The Stress Less Workbook

The Stress Less Workbook

Simple Strategies to Relieve Pressure,
Manage Commitments, and Minimize Conflicts

JONATHAN S. ABRAMOWITZ, PhD

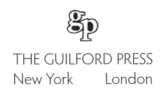

THE GUILFORD PRESS
New York   London

© 2012 The Guilford Press
A Division of Guilford Publications, Inc.
72 Spring Street, New York, NY 10012
www.guilford.com

Printed in the United States of America

This book is printed on acid-free paper.

Last digit is print number: 9   8   7   6   5   4   3   2   1

Library of Congress Cataloging-in-Publication Data

Abramowitz, Jonathan S.
   The stress less workbook : simple strategies to relieve pressure, manage commitments, and minimize conflicts / Jonathan S. Abramowitz. — 1st ed.
       p.   cm.
   Includes bibliographical references and index.
   ISBN 978-1-60918-471-1 (pbk. : alk. paper)
   1. Stress (Psychology)   2. Stress management.   3. Cognitive therapy.   I. Title.
   BF575.S75A27 2012
   155.9′042—dc23
                                                                        2012013195

To my loving and supportive parents,
Ferne and Leslie Abramowitz,
who taught me that
what doesn't kill us makes us stronger

Contents

Part I

Stress: Familiar to Us All but Understood by Few

Part II

Reducing Your Stress

Part III

Making Stress Management Techniques Work in Your Daily Life

Acknowledgments

Writing the Acknowledgments section is one of the great perks of writing a book—I'd almost equate it with giving an acceptance speech at the Academy Awards, where winners thank the most influential people in their lives. It would be nice if everyone could, at some point in life, take part in this custom because it's a wonderful tradition as well as a great stress-reduction technique. Research demonstrates that showing appreciation is related to being happier and more satisfied with life. People who express their gratitude feel more physically healthy, spend more time exercising, and experience less envy and other negative emotions. After all, when you're grateful for what you have, you're not obsessed with wanting more. And when you appreciate other people, it's hard to feel bad about them.

So, I am pleased to begin with my most influential teachers—Kathy Harring, T. Joel Wade, Art Houts, Edna Foa, Marty Franklin, and Michael Kozak—who taught me to appreciate psychology as a science. Yet much of what I've learned about stress, stress management, and other topics in behavioral health came while shivering through 6 years working at the Mayo Clinic in Rochester, Minnesota, with Kristi Dahlmann, Jill Snugeruud, Sarah Kalsy, Karen Grazier, Sheila Wadewicz, Matt Clark, Donald Williams, and Kristin Vickers-Douglass. Their insights can be found weaving in and out of the pages of this book.

And then comes Chris Benton, my editor and critic, with so much talent and patience. She read my drafts, understood my message, and helped me say what I wanted to say with the perfect blend of constructive feedback and positive reinforcement. She was my conscience as I wrote. Thanks also to Kitty Moore of The Guilford Press and Martin Antony, series editor, both of whom encouraged me to write this book and helped guide its structure.

Last, but certainly not least, I couldn't ask for a better form of stress management than my adoring wife and best friend, Stacy, and our terrific girls, Emily and Miriam. In every way possible, they supported me and my writing (sometimes even giving me the opportunity to practice my own stress-reduction skills). Thank you for your inspiration, understanding, and sacrifices while I worked on this project. To me, your love and happiness are the most important things in the world.

I have poured my heart and soul into these pages, and now I hope that my words will touch your mind and body.

Introduction

Do you get stressed out at work, at home, in social situations, or in other areas of your life? Maybe your doctor has warned you about potentially serious medical consequences if you don't learn ways of reducing stress. Maybe you're starting to notice that stress is robbing you of energy and focus, giving you a recurring headache or stiff neck, or harming your important relationships as you struggle to keep irritability and exhaustion out of your interactions with family, coworkers, friends, and even strangers. You may have picked up this book because you know you can't go on like this much longer. But you may also be worried about what you might be getting yourself into. A *workbook*? Isn't more work likely to just *add* to your stress?

The answer to that critical question is no. The book you're about to read involves work mainly in the sense that it allows you to work your way through identifying and resolving or reducing the stresses in your life one simple step at a time. One of the ironies of being overstressed is that it's easy to make things worse as you lose valuable sleep trying to figure out what you need to do to relieve the pressure. Before you know it, you're tangled up in stress imposed not just from the outside but from the inside too, as you try in vain to come up with solutions and then berate yourself when you can't.

This book offers an alternative: a *stress-less* way out of the trap so many of us find ourselves in. Not only will it help you accurately identify what's really exerting the pressure, but it will help you then chart a realistic course toward *less* stress. I won't promise you'll end up with *no* stress (which is unrealistic and also unwise since some stress is necessary to get us to important goals), but you will end up with less—so that you can reclaim your health, your productivity, and your enjoyment of all the best things life has to offer. That's because besides giving you a wealth of strategies to choose from, this book also shows you how to apply them in the typically stressful situations that we all encounter at some time or another. Let's face it: There are stressors you can eliminate and stressors you're stuck with. This book will help you reduce the negative impact of both.

Working through this book should be a fulfilling yet challenging experience. *Ful-

filling because the skills you learn will probably help you improve many areas of your life. Imagine reducing your risk of heart attack or stroke, sleeping better, being able to manage your time more effectively, having fewer anger outbursts, and feeling confident about solving problems. Imagine less pressure at holiday time and feeling like you're relaxed and able to live in the moment. Sounds nice, doesn't it?

This workbook will also be *challenging* because learning the skills to achieve these goals requires practice. Have you tried stress management programs before? Maybe you didn't get the results you wanted. Are you currently seeing a professional? Maybe it's difficult to find someone who really knows how to help you deal with the stressful situations in your life. Perhaps you've thought about getting help but haven't actually done so. Many people never recognize how stressed out they are until it's too late—the damage has been done—which is one of the main reasons I've written this book.

This may be your first attempt to do anything about stress. Whatever the case may be, by picking up this workbook you've chosen a program that has plenty of scientific research behind it. I've worked with hundreds of people to help them manage their stress. So I understand the nature of stress and how to treat it. In writing this book I've drawn on my knowledge of the research literature, as well as my clinical expertise, to make the most effective techniques for stress accessible to you in the most user-friendly format available. Basically, I have taken the strategies that are proven to be useful in therapy and adapted them in a self-help format for you. I will be your coach—teaching you all the tricks of the trade to help you overcome this problem. I will also be your cheerleader—giving you the encouragement you need to persevere.

WHO AM I?

Like most people, I'm no stranger to experiencing stress—after all, I survived 4 years of college, 7 years of graduate school and postgraduate training, and now I have a wife and two daughters! But when I was working as a psychologist at the Mayo Clinic (from 2000 through 2006), I got to observe firsthand how too much stress plays a role in problems such as obesity, cancer, heart disease, and other serious ailments. The physicians at Mayo understood this too, and they routinely referred their patients to our team for psychological evaluation. When we developed a stress management program, these physicians were eager to have us work with their patients; and they frequently told us how much our program contributed to helping patients manage and overcome their medical problems.

I am now Professor and Associate Chair of the Department of Psychology at the University of North Carolina (UNC) at Chapel Hill. I'm also director of the UNC Anxiety and Stress Disorders Clinic—an outpatient program that provides state-of-the-art psychological treatments for people with these problems. In addition to doing therapy with my own patients, I train and supervise PhD students—the psychologists of tomorrow—in how to understand, study, and use effective treatments for stress and anxiety. Our team also conducts research on prevention and treatment so that we can minimize the physical and mental suffering associated with these problems.

I love my work, but what's most rewarding to me is helping people like you apply the principles and techniques illustrated in this workbook to reduce the negative influence of stress and anxiety in their lives—whether it's to help treat or prevent a medical or psychological problem or just improve your quality of life. Given my interest in and love of this work, and the extraordinary training and experience I've been so fortunate to have as a clinician and a scientist, writing *The Stress Less Workbook* seemed like the obvious thing to do for all the people that I can't work with face to face. I hope you'll find that this book contains everything that our field has to offer.

HOW CAN THIS WORKBOOK HELP YOU?

In my work with patients and in my research, one thing has become very clear: each of us responds a little differently to stressful situations. That's why I'll teach you many different techniques for managing stress. You'll probably find that some work better for you than others; but most of them fall under the broad category of cognitive-behavioral therapy (CBT). CBT is an active, hands-on, skills-based approach to making changes in your life. I encourage you to have a pencil or pen handy as you read and to make copies of the blank worksheets and forms for your personal use so you can continue to use them even after you've completed reading the book.

This is a self-help book—meaning it's designed for you to use on your own—but it's not intended to *replace* treatment by a qualified mental health practitioner should you need professional help. You can use this book in any of these ways:

- *As a supplement to working with a therapist.* In fact, one of my motives for writing this book was to have a good resource for my own patients and clients to use as they progress through treatment. If you've tried therapy without much success, it may be that your therapist is not a specialist in the treatment of stress. If you've found a clinician that you like and trust—a critical ingredient in effective therapy—you may want to share this book to enrich the therapeutic relationship, giving you and your therapist a common language and common goals. As a companion to your treatment, this workbook can move your therapy forward and give it some structure.

- *For help with stress that does not require ongoing professional care.* One reason that many people do not get professional help for problems with stress is that they've found ways to live with it. That doesn't mean, however, that their lives aren't impaired—or that they could not benefit from improvement. In the chapters of Part I I'll help you get a feel for the severity of your stress, how it's affecting you, and whether you should see a mental health professional for a diagnostic evaluation. If not, self-directed treatment with this workbook may very well be appropriate for you. ***If you're feeling depressed or having thoughts about suicide, of course you should see a doctor right away.***

- *If you have problems with stress and are looking for more emotional support.* The stories and examples you will read here—composites of real people (whose identities are carefully disguised to protect their confidentiality), real symptoms, and real victories I have witnessed—will help you see that you are not alone in your struggle to gain better control over stress. The people I counsel often feel ashamed of how much—and the different ways—their lives are impacted by stress, *despite the fact that they are not to blame.* Shame and guilt are obstacles to self-improvement that get swept away the more you see that problems with stress come uninvited into innocent people's lives.

- *To facilitate your support network.* This workbook can help your friends, family members, and mental health professionals gain a fuller knowledge of how stress affects you, better understand what you are going through, and learn some tools for helping you manage your problems.

WHAT'S INSIDE?

Do you have mixed feelings about starting a stress management program? On one hand, you feel stuck; but on the other, change can produce even more stress. You'd like to be able to deal with difficult situations in your life more effectively, but what will it take? With all of these mixed emotions, you might be feeling confused and vulnerable. The strategies in this book will empower you by helping you understand your feelings better. I'll also help you get beyond the stress that's probably keeping you stuck right now.

This workbook is divided into three parts. Part I, which contains Chapters 1, 2, 3, and 4, will help you learn about stress, how it's affecting you, and what you can do about it. Stress can be triggered by lots of different situations; and in Part I, I'll help you learn more about your particular "stressors" so you can build a stress management program to meet your specific needs. Part II then teaches you the nuts and bolts of seven techniques proven to help reduce stress: problem solving (Chapter 5), effective communication (Chapter 6), time management (Chapter 7), cognitive therapy (Chapter 8), relaxation and meditation (Chapter 9), and maintaining healthy living behaviors (Chapter 10). In-depth descriptions, worksheets, and numerous examples provide you with step-by-step instructions for how to use each approach. In Part III, I then show you how to take the seven stress management techniques and apply them to three areas where it's common to experience stress: at work (Chapter 11), in your relationships and family (Chapter 12), and when a crisis hits (Chapter 13). The final chapter in this section (Chapter 14) focuses on helping you incorporate what you've learned into a "stress-less lifestyle" that will increase your lifetime resilience to the effects of stressful situations.

Now that you know what's in store, it's time to get started. Chapter 1 begins your passage toward a "stress-less" life—one with less emotional and physical turmoil and more serenity, success, and satisfaction.

Part I

Stress:
Familiar to Us All
but Understood by Few

1

How Stressed Out Are You?

Austin seemed to have it all. He owned a profitable business, had a terrific family, and lived in a lovely home. But Austin was a perfectionist, and it was making him miserable. He would get to work at the crack of dawn and stay late into the night, but still never seemed to get enough done. On most days he had headaches, felt fatigued, and had difficulty concentrating. Austin got angry very easily. He would yell at his wife and kids so much that they stopped including him in family activities. Each day brought new frustrations. Nothing made Austin happy—not his business, not his family, not his new sports car, and certainly not himself. Then, when his wife began talking about separating, Austin realized that he was upsetting everyone who was important to him and risking everything he valued. He was suffering from too much stress and it was wrecking his life.

Sharon and her husband, Nick, were high school sweethearts. They settled in their hometown, got married, and had children. But when Nick's company transferred him to a new city, they had to move a very long way. That's when things started to go downhill for Sharon. She wasn't the same person she had been before the move. Her stomach felt queasy all the time. She didn't feel like eating or being intimate with Nick. She was tense and couldn't sleep well. And she worried a lot about making friends in her new city. She spent a lot of time by herself, often calling her old friends to complain about being so far away from her hometown. A few months later, Sharon noticed that her husband was enjoying his new job. And the kids were happy in their new school. But Sharon was missing out. Her stress had prevented her from getting on with her new life.

Austin and Sharon are not alone. In fact, everyone knows the feeling that we call "stress." Modern life, after all, is full of stressful events: pressures, frustrations, hassles, demands, deadlines, aggravations, annoyances, interruptions, and the like. Stressful events vary tremendously from minor irritations to major life-changing experiences. You're late for an important meeting. The car won't start. You're having trouble at work. You fail an exam or bomb an important assignment. You argue with a close friend or relative. You separate or divorce from a romantic partner. Someone you love is very ill or even dying.

Although we usually think of negative events as creating stress, stress can also occur when positive events have a major impact on you. For example, you start a new job, get promoted, get married, have a new baby, or win an important award. The Eye Opener below lists the most stressful events according to research studies.

Feelings of stress vary in their intensity from a brief, almost fleeting flash, to constant worrying, to all-out panic. For some people, stress is so chronic that it becomes a way of life. If you frequently find yourself feeling tense, overwhelmed, and frazzled, it's time you took action. It turns out that learning and practicing some straightforward skills and techniques is the key to managing stress so that stress doesn't end up managing you. But as you'll see, stress is complex. It's multifaceted. And not surprisingly, it affects everyone a little differently. So, successfully managing your own stress begins with understanding what it is, how it's affecting you, and what you can do about it. And that's just what we'll do to start things off in this workbook. Noted stress researcher Hans Selye once said that stress is "too well known and too little understood." So, in this first chapter, we'll begin by examining your current stress levels and what's happening in your body when you feel stress. We'll also explore *why* you have stress in the first place—and some of this might surprise you.

HOW STRESSED ARE YOU?

To determine your current stress level, fill out the Perceived Stress Scale on the facing page. This is a scale you'll want to complete every month or so to monitor how you're doing with reducing stress; so you might make copies for future use. For each question, mark an "X" next to the number that corresponds to how often you have each thought

---

EYE OPENER

Top 10 Stressful Life Events

1. Spouse's death
2. Divorce
3. Marriage separation
4. Serving time in jail
5. Close relative's death
6. Serious illness or injury
7. Getting married
8. Being fired from a job
9. Marriage reconciliation
10. Retirement

PERCEIVED STRESS SCALE

1. In the last month, how often have you been upset because of something that happened unexpectedly?
   _____ 0 = never
   _____ 1 = almost never
   _____ 2 = sometimes
   _____ 3 = fairly often
   _____ 4 = very often

2. In the last month, how often have you felt that you were unable to control the important things in your life?
   _____ 0 = never
   _____ 1 = almost never
   _____ 2 = sometimes
   _____ 3 = fairly often
   _____ 4 = very often

3. In the last month, how often have you felt nervous and "stressed"?
   _____ 0 = never
   _____ 1 = almost never
   _____ 2 = sometimes
   _____ 3 = fairly often
   _____ 4 = very often

4. In the last month, how often have you felt confident about your ability to handle your personal problems?
   _____ 4 = never
   _____ 3 = almost never
   _____ 2 = sometimes
   _____ 1 = fairly often
   _____ 0 = very often

5. In the last month, how often have you felt that things were going your way?
   _____ 4 = never
   _____ 3 = almost never
   _____ 2 = sometimes
   _____ 1 = fairly often
   _____ 0 = very often

6. In the last month, how often have you found that you could not cope with all the things that you had to do?
   _____ 0 = never
   _____ 1 = almost never
   _____ 2 = sometimes
   _____ 3 = fairly often
   _____ 4 = very often

7. In the last month, how often have you been able to control irritations in your life?
   _____ 4 = never
   _____ 3 = almost never
   _____ 2 = sometimes
   _____ 1 = fairly often
   _____ 0 = very often

8. In the last month, how often have you felt that you were on top of things?
   _____ 4 = never
   _____ 3 = almost never
   _____ 2 = sometimes
   _____ 1 = fairly often
   _____ 0 = very often

9. In the last month, how often have you been angered because of things that were outside of your control?
   _____ 0 = never
   _____ 1 = almost never
   _____ 2 = sometimes
   _____ 3 = fairly often
   _____ 4 = very often

10. In the last month, how often have you felt difficulties were piling up so high that you could not overcome them?
    _____ 0 = never
    _____ 1 = almost never
    _____ 2 = sometimes
    _____ 3 = fairly often
    _____ 4 = very often

Adapted with permission from Cohen, S., Kamarck, T., and Mermelstein, R. (1983). A global measure of perceived stress. *Journal of Health and Social Behavior, 24,* 385–396. Copyright 1983 by the American Sociological Association.

Reprinted in *The Stress Less Workbook.* Copyright 2012 by The Guilford Press.

or feeling. You'll get the most benefit from this exercise if you use a pencil or pen and write your answers down, rather than just thinking about them or "doing it in your head." There's something about writing that forces you to think more clearly and carefully about your answers.

Now, calculate your total score by adding up the numbers next to where you marked your "X" for each question (notice that for some of the questions the numbering is reversed). The highest possible score you can have is 40. Enter your score below:

Perceived Stress Scale Total Score = _____

What does your score mean? If your total score is 15 or less, either you haven't experienced too many stressful events lately or you're managing the pressures, demands, and hassles of everyday life reasonably well. If so, good for you! You'll find the techniques in this workbook helpful for perfecting your already well-honed stress-busting skills.

If your score is between 16 and 25, you're probably experiencing at least a moderate degree of stress in your life. Maybe you can manage your stressful circumstances some of the time; but at other times they get the best of you. Perhaps you've experienced some major life changes that have thrown you for a loop. Think about work (or school), your personal life and relationships, and your health—your stress is likely to come from these sources. Has life become very demanding? Does it seem like you don't have enough time to do everything you want to (or *have* to)? Luckily, you can use the strategies in this book to help you reduce much of the stress in your life and deal effectively with that which remains. Read on!

If your score is 26 or above, you're probably dealing with a great deal of stress on a daily basis. You might be having trouble managing important unpredictable or uncontrollable events in your life. Or perhaps it's that lots of everyday hassles and pressures are adding up and making you feel overwhelmed. You might feel tired and fatigued. Maybe your fuse is short these days. Life is probably less enjoyable than it has been—or could be. If so, to gain the upper hand and take charge, you should work through the exercises in this book thoughtfully and carefully—perhaps even with a professional. Problems such as anxiety, depression, and anger often accompany severe stress. In Chapter 2 we'll look at these issues more closely and determine whether it might be a good idea to seek professional help.

Finally, stress can be hard to perceive when you're right in the middle of it. It takes its toll on your mind and body before you even realize it's there. In Chapter 2 you'll learn about the longer-term cumulative effects of stress. So, even if your score on the preceding scale isn't very high, you'll want to read Chapter 2 before you decide that your stress level is lower than you thought when you picked up this book.

WHAT IS STRESS?

No matter what your score is on the Perceived Stress Scale, it's important to remember that everyone (yes, *everyone*) experiences at least *some* stress from time to time. Stress is universal—it occurs in all cultures around the world. It's a normal part of being human. But what exactly *is* stress? To gain the upper hand on this complex enemy you'll need to understand its workings.

The best way of thinking about stress is that it is the body's way of responding to events and situations that upset your balance or make you feel threatened in one way or another. In short, it's a state of readiness. When you sense danger—whether the danger is real or just imagined—your body automatically rises to the occasion and prepares you to take action and protect yourself.

A *stressor*, then, is any event, situation, condition, or demand that causes you stress by disrupting your life balance in some way. Life is full of challenges that may be considered stressors. In fact, you could think of any change in your regular lifestyle or routine as a stressor. Obvious examples include the events listed in the Eye Opener on page 8. Less-well-known examples include exposure to loud noise, extreme heat or cold, and personal issues such as questioning your core values, sense of purpose, or future plans. Your own illnesses and injuries also qualify as stressors, as do arguments with friends. As I mentioned before, even positive events—getting married, starting a new job, celebrating an important milestone or significant award—can be stressors. In Chapter 3, I'll help you identify *your* stressors—those situations that may be disrupting your balance and causing you to feel stress.

Perception Is Everything

How stressed out you feel at a given time depends on how much you perceive yourself as under the gun. If you view a particular stressor as only mildly or somewhat problematic, your stress level may only be low to moderate. But when you view it as catastrophic or overwhelming, or if you see yourself as being unable to cope, your level of stress skyrockets! So, being late to a lunch date with friends may trigger only a little stress. Being late for a business lunch with an important client triggers a whole lot more. We'll come back to this important point in Chapter 8. It turns out that since our thoughts and perceptions have so much to do with how much stress we experience, one important strategy for managing stress involves developing more useful ways of thinking about stressors.

Stress is what you experience when you perceive a threat, have demands placed on you, or are exposed to extreme or distressing conditions.

What's Good about Stress?

Stress probably seems like something you could do without, right? It can feel very uncomfortable (perhaps painful). It can disrupt your relationships. It can lead to bad habits such as overeating and smoking. And it may ultimately make you more vulnerable to serious medical problems such as heart disease. But ask yourself this question: could stress *ever* be a good thing?

Yes, it can. Believe it or not, your stress response is actually a fundamentally help-

The Fight-or-Flight Response Isn't Just for Humans

Humans are not the only animals that have a fight-or-flight response. In fact, virtually all members of the animal kingdom—right down to the sea slug—have this response. Even our pets can feel stressed. And not just dogs and cats. Stress responses have been found in birds, fish, and even hamsters and guinea pigs.

ful, adaptive, life-sustaining, even crucial system of your body. Having stress is neither a personal weakness nor a mental illness. Remember when I said stress is intended to get you ready to protect yourself from danger? Eons ago when humans lived in the wild with other animals (including predators), having an automatic response take over when danger arose—for instance, an approaching saber-toothed tiger—was critical to self-preservation. This stress response, often called the *fight-or-flight response*, prepares us instantly to either fight back or run for our lives. The fight-or-flight response is a dramatic series of changes that we'll explore more fully in the next section. This automatic response ensured that prehistoric humans would survive in an otherwise dangerous environment. Clearly it was beneficial to our forebears. But what has it done for us lately?

Stress in Modern Times

Despite the fact that our fiercest predators are no longer an ever-present threat, we still need our stress response from time to time. Imagine that you're crossing the street, but there's a car speeding toward you, blasting its horn. If you didn't have a stress response, you'd probably be killed! Luckily, however, your body's fight-or-flight response automatically takes over and pushes you out of harm's way.

Fortunately, in today's modern world, life-threatening stressors are relatively few and far between. Of course, we're not totally out of the woods—modern life still has its share of potentially dangerous situations. Depending on where you live, you might face a threat of violent crime, terrorist attacks, severe weather (such as hurricanes), or natural disasters (such as earthquakes). And occasionally we all hear about dangers associated with driving, swimming, and fire. For the most part, though, the near constant physical dangers of prehistoric times have been replaced by social and psychological stressors of modern life that come from work or school, relationships, finances, your health, and even daily life hassles.

These modern-day stressors may not pose the same kind of threat to life and limb as our ancestors faced, but your body doesn't know how to tell the difference. To your brain and the rest of your body, *a threat is a threat*. So, to be on the safe side, it reacts the same way it did when your ancestors faced life-threatening dangers. Just think of yourself taking an exam when it dawns on you that you studied the wrong material! As you look over the questions, you realize that you don't know the answers and will fail the test. In today's world, it's tests, traffic, relationships, computers and other machines, office politics, daily hassles, and the like that are most likely to trigger stress. Although generally less physically threatening than the dangers of old, these stressors still provoke the same intense response.

COMPONENTS OF THE STRESS RESPONSE

Your stress response is highly complex. In this chapter we'll deal with the *immediate* effects of stress—that is, what happens to your body right as you notice yourself becoming stressed out. In Chapter 2, you'll learn about how your body is affected by experiencing stress over the long term.

The immediate stress response is made up of three types of reactions, all of which are geared primarily to helping you cope with danger and keeping you out of harm's way. We're going to explore these three reactions in some detail because understanding exactly what's happening to you when you become stressed is an important step in taking charge of stress. The three reactions are:

- *Physical reactions*, which can include sweating, greater muscle tension, nausea, an increased breathing rate, and a racing heart.

- *Mental reactions*, which include a shift in attention and racing thoughts about the possible outcomes of a situation.

- *Behavioral reactions*, which may include anger, hostility, perfectionism, and the urge to escape.

Physical Reactions to Stress

The physical component of stress is often the most noticeable, so let's start there. Check the box next to each of the physical reactions that you notice when you feel stressed:

- ❑ Increased breathing or difficulty catching your breath
- ❑ Racing or pounding heart
- ❑ Pain or discomfort in the chest or elsewhere
- ❑ Hot or cold flashes
- ❑ Dry mouth (less saliva)
- ❑ Nausea or stomach distress
- ❑ Loss of appetite
- ❑ Sweating

❑ Muscle tension

❑ Trembling or shaking

❑ Unsteadiness, dizziness, or feeling faint

❑ Numbness or tingling in your arms, fingers, legs, or toes

❑ Feelings of "unreality" or "derealization"

❑ Dilated pupils, leading to blurry vision or spots

Although these reactions sometimes feel very intense, uncontrollable, and uncomfortable (they might even seem very scary—like you're having a panic attack, losing control, or having a medical emergency), they are all part of your body's normal stress response. And your body knows what it's doing! Believe it or not, all of these physical sensations play a role in keeping you safe. Read on to find out how.

When you encounter a stressful situation and perceive danger or threat, your brain sends messages to a part of your nervous system called the *autonomic nervous system*. The autonomic nervous system—which has two branches: the *sympathetic* and *parasympathetic* branches—is involved in directly controlling the body's energy levels and preparation for action. It's the *sympathetic* branch that releases energy and primes your body for action by causing the physical responses listed above. The *parasympathetic* branch, on the other hand, is responsible for restoring your body to a normal state (sometimes called the *rest-and-digest* response).

Sympathetic Nervous System

The sympathetic nervous system releases two chemicals, adrenaline and noradrenaline, from the adrenal glands of the kidneys. Energized by these two chemicals, the stress response (and the related physical reactions) can continue for quite some time. Activation of the sympathetic nervous system increases your heart rate and strength of your heartbeat, your breathing rate, and blood flow throughout your body. This is important for survival because blood provides your muscles with the nutrients they might need to help you fight or run away from danger. Like a reflex, the sympathetic nervous system automatically directs blood away from places where it is not needed (such as your fingers and toes), by tightening the blood vessels, and toward places where it is needed more (such as the large muscles in your arms and legs), by expanding those blood vessels.

The increased breathing rate that you experience during stress helps ensure that the blood pumping through your body is rich with oxygen. Your muscles use this oxygen to produce energy. Yet the high rate of breathing can cause chest pains and even produce feelings of choking or suffocating—like you can't get enough air. Temporary feelings such as confusion, dizziness, "unreality," and even blurred vision can also result from the changes in breathing rate and the automatic dilation of your pupils (to let in more light in case it is night). But rest assured that these sensations are only temporary. They go away when your body returns to a resting state.

The Eye Opener on the next page summarizes what happens when the sympathetic nervous system is activated, which actually affects most systems of the body. These reactions require lots of energy, so it is common for you to feel drained at the end of a stressful day. But be assured that your body won't get carried away or "out of control." And even intense bursts of stress will not harm you (physically or mentally). After all, remember that the purpose of the fight-or-flight response is to *protect* you from harm and keep you safe. It wouldn't make any sense for us to have a protective response that then turns around and double-crosses us by causing harm.

Parasympathetic Nervous System

The reason you don't have to worry about your stress response raging on forever, getting out of control, or leading to a "breakdown" is that your parasympathetic nervous system eventually steps in and keeps things in check. After the perceived threat has passed, or after enough time has gone by, this system takes over and restores a calmer state by breaking down the adrenaline and noradrenaline in your bloodstream. Sometimes this process seems to take longer than you would like. But rest assured that it *will* happen. In the meantime, you'll probably feel a little jumpy, jittery, or edgy for a while. This is normal even *after* you've dealt with whatever triggered your stress in the first place. Adrenaline and noradrenaline can take some time to be broken down; and that's a holdover from ancient times when dangerous animals would return over and over to stalk humans. So, staying keyed up for a while after noticing a predator probably helped ensure the survival of our earliest ancestors.

Mental and Emotional Reactions to Stress

Check the box next to each of the mental or emotional reactions that you notice when you feel stressed:

- ❏ Being preoccupied with what's stressing you out
- ❏ Thinking of the worst possible outcome
- ❏ Predicting that bad things will happen
- ❏ Second-guessing yourself
- ❏ Having racing thoughts
- ❏ Problems with your memory
- ❏ Difficulty concentrating on things
- ❏ Being easily distractible
- ❏ Trouble paying attention
- ❏ Feeling overwhelmed

Effects of the Sympathetic Nervous System

When you perceive a threat and your sympathetic nervous system becomes active, your body undergoes a wide range of changes, all of which are designed to help you respond to possible danger by fighting or fleeing. Here are the most commonly noticed body changes and their purpose:

Physical reaction	Purpose
• Increased heart rate	Circulates blood to your body's large muscles
• Increased breathing	Gets more oxygen (energy) into your body
• Sweating	Cools your body to keep it from overheating
• Stomach discomfort/nausea	Keeps you from feeling hungry
• Muscle tension/tremors	Keeps you alert and ready to fight or run
• Easy to startle	Keeps you ready to respond to physical threat
• Pupils dilate or widen	Lets more light in so you can see in the dark

When feeling stressed, you might also notice the symptoms listed below. Although these might feel uncomfortable or seem scary, rest assured that they are part of the normal stress response.

Symptom	Explanation
• Exhaustion/fatigue	The stress reaction requires a great deal of energy, so it is normal to feel tired and drained during times of high stress.
• Hot flash/flushed	Blood is directed to the large muscles in the core of your body, which makes you feel hot.
• Cold or clammy hands	Blood is directed away from your hands, so they may appear white and feel cold.
• Numb/tingling in extremities	Blood is directed away from these areas, almost like your hands and feet are "falling asleep."
• Aches or pain	This results from prolonged muscle tension.
• Constipation	This results from reduced digestive system activity.
• Blurred vision or seeing spots	This results from dilated pupils.
• Dizziness/faintness/unreality	This is temporary and results from the rapid increase in your breathing rate.

❑ Worrying

❑ Feeling irritable

Imagine living in prehistoric times when you constantly had to be on the lookout for potential danger. If you let down your guard even for a moment, you might end up becoming a meal for a predator. The mental part of the stress response is a holdover from those bygone days when the human mind was used primarily to survive in such a dangerous environment.

Shifts in Attention and Alertness

What good is a fight-or-flight response if you can't tell when danger is present? That's why when you become stressed, the focus of your attention automatically shifts. You instinctively go on high alert, scanning your surroundings and analyzing the situation to look for any warning signs of trouble. You become preoccupied with the stressor. This shift in attention and hyperalertness is useful to the extent that it helps you quickly recognize any dangers that might be present. Thank goodness our ancestors had this innate response—survival of the human race probably depended on it way back then (this also explains why stress is associated with sleep loss—*if you snooze, you lose*).

Although truly life-threatening dangers are few and far between in today's modern world, the human mind still reacts to a perceived threat the same way it did in prehistoric times. And because we now use our minds for many tasks other than staying alive, when you become preoccupied with a stressor, it's going to sap your brain of the mental energy that you'd otherwise use for things such as paying attention in a conversation, learning and memorizing facts in school, focusing and concentrating on a task at work, and thinking logically about how to solve a problem. It's almost like there's a game of tug-of-war going on in your brain: the stressful situation is (for the time being) trying to tug your attention and concentration away from all your other daily concerns. Because the stressful situation is a source of *threat*, the other daily matters don't stand a chance. Here are some ways the tug-of-war game may affect your mental energy.

- When you're stressed, you might find it hard to concentrate on anything other than what's stressing you out. Like a computer, your brain has only so many resources. When an important stressor steals a lot of your mental energy, there is less available for other tasks.

- You might become totally preoccupied or "obsessed" with the situation you're stressed about. That's because your mind is automatically giving this situation the highest priority. It's scanning and preparing for a possible threat.

- You might also be easily distracted if you are talking to someone, or trying to work, read, or watch TV. Again that's your stress response instinctively reminding you about a potential threat.

- As I mentioned earlier, you might have trouble falling asleep because your body wants to stay on high alert (it thinks danger could be lurking).

- The tug-of-war game also explains why you might seem to have memory problems when under a lot of stress. *But there's actually nothing wrong with your memory.* It's just that most of your mind's resources are *temporarily* being used up to deal with the potentially threatening situation. Your memory will come back later.

Worrying

One of the things your mind automatically does when it is stressed is try to consider many possible outcomes of the stressful or threatening situation. You sort through all the awful things that could happen to you or to the people you care about. This type of "catastrophic thinking" is called *worrying*. It's the brain's way of ensuring that nothing can take you by surprise—an important advantage for prehistoric humans, although nowadays worrying usually creates more distress than it prevents. Imagine that an important project at work isn't going so well. You feel stressed and start thinking how the boss will respond. Will you get a negative evaluation? Will it affect your salary or that promotion you were hoping for? Could you even be fired? Will you be able to find another job? How will you support your family? What will your friends and family think? When you feel bothered or troubled about a stressor and you can't seem to get your mind off it, you're probably worrying.

Of course, everyone worries from time to time. It's normal . . . up to a point. Another name for normal worrying is being *concerned*. Concern is useful. It reminds us how important something is. It keeps us levelheaded and helps us solve our problems effectively. For example, "This project isn't going so well. Maybe I should talk with the boss and fill her in so we can figure out how to get things back on track." When your concerns escalate into worries, that's when problems begin. Uncontrollable racing thoughts about dreaded, awful, or catastrophic outcomes (for example, "Oh no! What will I do when I get fired!?") might consume your day, keep you from being able to accomplish things you want to accomplish, and interfere with your sleep, appetite, and sex drive. Yes, worrying too much actually gets in the way of solving problems! Fortunately, you can use the techniques in this workbook to rein in unproductive worrisome thoughts and revamp them into healthy concerns that will motivate you to solve problems and cope effectively.

Behavioral Reactions

The following checklist includes behaviors that people often do when they feel stressed. Place a check mark next to those that you notice. You might also have someone who knows you well go through the checklist because sometimes when we're under stress we aren't fully aware of our own behavior:

❒ Snapping at people

❒ Starting arguments

❒ Starting physical fights

❒ Destroying property

❒ Pacing

❒ Tapping your feet or fingers

❒ Biting your nails

❒ Picking your skin or pulling your hair

❒ Using alcohol

❒ Using drugs

❒ Smoking

❒ Snacking on "comfort foods"

❒ Avoiding people or situations

The fight-or-flight response gets its name from the fact that its number-one purpose is to prepare you for *action*—attacking or fleeing to safety. So, it shouldn't be surprising that stress is associated with the buildup of nervous energy and the overwhelming urge to release this energy by being aggressive or trying to escape from wherever you are. Do you become angry, hostile, or even violent when you're under a great deal of stress? Have you ever punched a wall, thrown or destroyed an object, or started a fight when you were feeling under the gun? Do people who are close to you tell you that you have anger problems? Maybe you can restrain yourself from acting destructively, but the aggressive urges might still sneak out in other ways—such as starting arguments, snapping at people, or intentionally saying nasty or sarcastic things. Even nervous habits such as pacing, tapping, skin picking, nail biting, and snacking can be considered socially acceptable ways of releasing this nervous energy. Other behaviors, such as escaping from (or simply avoiding) unpleasant or stressful situations, are also part of this response.

Some behavior patterns that are motivated by stress, such as anger problems, smoking, and abusing alcohol and drugs, can be extremely destructive. Others, such as nail biting and skin picking, are generally less harmful as long as they occur in moderation. But even these simple behaviors can become habits that interfere with your enjoyment of life.

STRESS: A TWO-SIDED COIN

It's easy to think of stress as dreadful. After all, it may feel painful, lead to problems in your life, cause weight gain, depression, and in some cases create serious long-term health problems (we'll get to this in Chapter 2). But hopefully you now understand what I alluded to earlier in this chapter—stress is fundamentally *good*. It's there to help us survive. Remember, also, that stress is universal. We all experience it on a regular basis. So, even the most successful stress management program will not take stress away completely. Rather, the goal is to reduce stress just enough that it becomes manageable for you. Luckily, it's only when stress gets out of control that it is worthy of the bad rap that it often gets. So, to end this chapter, let's focus on some of the positive aspects of stress—some of the ways that normal levels of stress can actually make you a happier, healthier person.

Your body is actually designed to deal very well with most of the stress you experience. The adrenaline release that comes with feeling stress can help you focus and think more clearly and provide you with an energy burst to help you perform better and achieve your goals. We see this very often in situations such as sporting events, school achievement, and many creative and social activities. The graph on the facing page shows the "Yerkes–Dodson curve." It's named after Harvard University scientists Robert Yerkes and John Dodson, who discovered that up to a point as stress levels increase, so does performance. If you're feeling absolutely no stress (for example, when you are bored or lethargic), the left part of the curve shows that performance levels are typically also low. There's no motivation to perform at your best. When stress levels are in the moderate range, however, performance is at its peak because the stress is helping to push you to excel. The right side of the curve shows that performance levels diminish again when you feel excessive levels of stress.

So, the goal is to get to the top of the performance curve—which means that there will be *some* stress in your life . . . the helpful kind. Let's imagine you have an important presentation at work or school coming up. Stress helps make sure you're ready for it. Stress drives you to put your best foot forward and do as good a job as you can. If you didn't become stressed *at all*, you may not be motivated to prepare for the presentation. You might oversleep, be too laid back, act or dress inappropriately, and come off as a poor speaker. If you're too stressed, you might not be able to focus on giving your

---

EYE PENER

Stress Is Like a Guitar String

The image of a guitar string can help remind you that a moderate amount of stress (not too *low*, not too *high*) is ideal for peak performance levels: When a guitar string is too loose (not enough tension), it plays notes that are too low (flat). And if there's no tension at all, it can't produce any sound. Similarly, if the string is strung too tightly (too much tension), it plays notes that are too high (sharp). Strings that are too tight will even snap. If the string, however, has just the right amount of tension, it results in perfect-sounding notes.

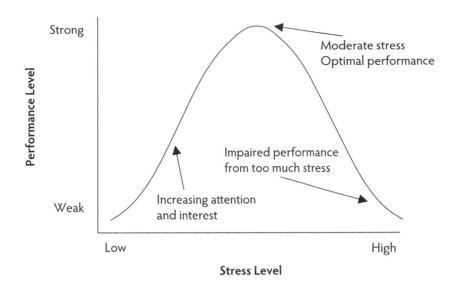

presentation because you're so wound up and worrying about how it will go. You might even forget the main points you need to tell your audience.

How Has Stress Helped You?

When I work with people suffering from stress-related problems, I ask them to think of ways in which their stress response might be (or has been) helpful for them. Here is some of what people have told me:

"As a writer, stress helps me be more creative." (Liam, novelist, age 42)

Ask any author or artist about the creative process and you'll hear that his or her best work comes as a result of a lot of head-pounding frustration and borderline agony. Stress often precedes or accompanies creative breakthroughs. Why? Because when you're totally calm and relaxed, you don't need a reason to be creative. It's stress that pushes you to be creative and think "outside the box."

"It's good for your immune system." (Bethany, medical doctor, age 52)

Research shows that the immune system benefits from short bursts of stress that elicit our fight-or-flight response. During short bursts of stress, cortisol (the "stress hormone") is released, which increases immunity in the body. Research also shows that experiencing short-term stress right before having surgery is actually associated with a speedier and more successful recovery. Of course, it's a delicate balance. While bursts of stress can keep your body strong and vibrant, too much of it over the long haul can lead to cortisol overload, which can cause weight gain and increase your chances of developing heart disease, diabetes, and having a stroke.

"It can help you get fit." (Michelle, fitness instructor, age 33)

Moderate exercise, such as lifting weights, running, or spending 45 sweaty minutes on the exercise bike, is a form of stress on your body. But it's the good kind of stress that we all know is very healthy. The demands that this type of stress puts on your body actually help you complete everyday activities more easily. Regular exercise also reduces levels of cortisol, while simultaneously increasing the level of endorphins, the natural chemicals in the body that produce feelings of well-being. In fact, research has shown that exercise itself may make us more resilient to the harmful effects of stress.

"It helps with problem solving." (Andrew, clinical psychologist, age 61)

When you're faced with a dilemma or a big decision, do you become *concerned*—a healthy type of stress—or do you *worry*, an unhealthy form? There's a delicate balance between these two, and while worry can actually get in the way of effective problem solving and decision making, an appropriate amount of *concern* can do a lot of good. That's because this type of stress helps us think about what's most important to us. It actually helps us care.

"It helps keep my kids safe." (Aaron, father, age 41)

Parents who feel more stress tend to keep their kids out of harm's way. That's because appropriate stress levels increase your alertness. Think about it: if you're concerned about kidnappers, you're more likely to keep a watchful eye on your child at the playground, right? Of course, being overly stressed out can lead to being hyperalert or hypervigilant, which interferes with child rearing because it can prevent the child from developing a healthy degree of independence.

"It may get you a raise." (Aliza, secretary, age 55)

Do you put in long hours at the office? Do you feel jumpy every time your boss walks into your cubicle? Sure, chronic job stress is bad for you. But the kind of stress that keeps you on your toes in your work environment is actually good for your career. As the Yerkes–Dodson curve shows, an optimal level of stress keeps you energized, focused, and motivated. You'll be performing at your peak. Without enough stress, you don't give your full effort and are more likely to make mistakes. Too much stress, on the other hand, saps your ability to see innovative solutions and takes a toll on your energy and efficiency.

Now it's your turn. To help you think about stress as a helpful, healthy experience, consider some ways that it has helped you out in life. Maybe it was something relatively trivial—deciding on which car to buy or which classes to take. Maybe stress helped you with "big-ticket" items such as deciding which job to take or planning a major event such as a wedding. Do you thrive under pressure? If so, you probably have lots of examples. Write down your answers in the spaces on the facing page.

_____

_____

_____

So, now you understand that stress is a normal, universal response to changes around us (that is, to *stressors*). Whether the change represents a possible threat, a demand, or some other alteration in your life, stress is there to help you cope. You've learned about the physical, mental, and behavioral responses that occur with stress—and how these responses are all geared toward keeping you safe and preparing you to take action. Finally, you've seen how not all stress is bad. In moderate amounts, it is beneficial in different areas of life. This workbook aims to help you get into that zone of moderate stress so that you can reach your peak potential. But if you are reading this, you probably have too much stress, and you probably experience it in ways that interfere with different aspects of your life (like the right side of the Yerkes–Dodson curve). Instead of the *short* bursts of stress, adrenaline, and cortisol that promote well-being, you might be suffering with the chronic and more severe form of stress. In Chapter 2 we'll focus on this darker side of stress. You'll learn about the negative effects that chronic stress can have and discover how it affects your everyday life. You'll also learn about the potentially devastating long-term effects of prolonged constant stress on your physical and mental health.

2

What Is Stress Doing to You?

As you learned in Chapter 1, stress, in small doses, is good for you. It makes you more alert and gives you a burst of energy. Remember that the fight-or-flight response and the related stress hormones affect many different parts of our bodies, from our muscles and tissues to our blood vessels and organs. The stress response temporarily speeds up many of the body's internal processes.

But the truth is that too much of this good thing will wreak havoc with your mind and body. That's because when you experience ongoing stress, your body doesn't have a chance to recuperate from the energy bursts. What's the result? Just like any other piece of machinery, when your body's organ systems are overused they begin to weaken and wear out, making you vulnerable to all sorts of medical and emotional problems. In fact, research shows that chronic stress can shorten life expectancy by 15 to 20 years. I don't mean to scare you, but *stress can kill.*

So, if you experience stress, then in one way or another it's taking a toll on you. Are you medically healthy? About half of people surveyed report that stress affects their physical well-being. Stress weakens your immune system, making you more vulnerable to infections and other kinds of ailments. Are you satisfied in your relationships with others? Nearly one in five people say that stress negatively impacts their marriage or friendships. How are things at school or work? About 15% of people say that their academic or job performance is affected by stress. One study found that on-the-job stress in the United States is responsible for absenteeism, lost productivity, accidents, and medical insurance costs totaling between $200 and $300 billion each year. These are sobering statistics.

How is stress affecting you? In this chapter we will look closely at the signs and symptoms of stress and examine how you're holding up mentally and physically. Keep in mind that stress has both *immediate* (short-term) and more *permanent* (long-term) effects. Fortunately, when you promptly recognize that you're under stress and take steps to reduce it, you can reverse the short-term effects. (And remember from Chapter 1 that a burst of stress courtesy of the fight-or-flight response is not going to kill you outright.) But if stress lingers on for months or years, the long-term effects may be irreversible.

Next, we'll look at what stress could do to you if you don't help yourself. We'll also help you to determine whether you'd be better off using this workbook along with some professional help.

WHAT ARE THE SIGNS AND SYMPTOMS OF STRESS?

In addition to the immediate effects created by the sympathetic nervous system discussed in Chapter 1, there is a wide array of *signs* (what a doctor notices during an examination) and *symptoms* (what you experience) of stress that range from mild and harmless feelings of tiredness or lethargy to life-threatening problems such as a heart attack or stroke. As you'd expect, the more serious problems occur when you experience lengthy periods of intense stress. These signs and symptoms belong to four categories: physical, mental, emotional, and behavioral. The chart below lists many of the signs and symptoms of stress. As you can see, these effects range from relatively minor to all-out life threatening.

Common Signs and Symptoms of Stress

Physical	Mental	Emotional	Behavioral
Headaches	Trouble concentrating	Anger	Overeating
Chest tightness	Forgetfulness	Anxiety	Fidgeting/nail biting
Tiredness/fatigue	Chronic worry	Depression	Trouble sleeping
Heart palpitations	Thoughts of death	Irritability	Loss of motivation and
Difficulty breathing	Indecisiveness	Guilt feelings	decreased activity
Constipation	Feeling helpless or	Overwhelmed	Irritability
Diarrhea	hopeless		Smoking
Heartburn/indigestion	Catastrophizing		Increased drug/alcohol
Loss of sex drive	(blowing things out of		use
Loss of appetite	proportion)		Crying
Excessive sweating			Increased caffeine use
Cardiovascular disease			Violence
Muscle spasms/cramps			Interpersonal conflict
Jaw pain			
Bruxism (grinding your teeth)			
Tremors and shakiness			
Chest pain			
Back pain			
Ulcers			
Muscle and joint pain			
Irritable bowel syndrome			
Rashes, hives, and other skin conditions			
Infections			
Arthritis			

HOW IS STRESS AFFECTING YOUR BODY?

Short-term stress has effects on almost every part of the body. Here are some common examples:

- The release of chemicals during the fight-or-flight response causes blood vessels in your brain to swell. The result: chronic tension headaches and migraines.

- Chronic stress suppresses the immune system, which makes it easier for you to get sick. Do you tend to cough and sneeze a lot when you've had a stressful week at work or school? This may be why.

- The chemicals released in your body during fight-or-flight trigger the sebaceous glands on your skin to produce more oil, leading to clogged pores and pimples.

Stress affects everyone differently. Some people have an intense response, while others may be only slightly affected. The following checklist contains 30 signs and symptoms that can be caused by stress. Put a check mark next to any you've experienced over the past month. Then put the total number of symptoms you've experienced in the blank at the bottom of the checklist.

- ❒ Cut
- ❒ Bruise
- ❒ Bloody nose
- ❒ Pimples
- ❒ Painful joints
- ❒ Muscle strain
- ❒ Eye strain
- ❒ Painful urination
- ❒ Headache
- ❒ Earache
- ❒ Toothache
- ❒ Chest pain
- ❒ Back pain
- ❒ Athlete's foot
- ❒ Nausea or vomiting
- ❒ Skin rash

❏ Diarrhea

❏ Constipation

❏ Indigestion

❏ Dizziness

❏ Sneezing

❏ Coughing

❏ Fatigue/tiredness during the day

❏ Loss of sex drive

❏ Allergy/hay fever

❏ Running nose

❏ Hoarse voice

❏ Sinus infection

❏ Asthma

❏ Shortness of breath

_____ **Total number of symptoms**

What was your score (how many check marks did you have)? Research shows that people who experience higher levels of stress tend to experience more of these symptoms. Of course, this doesn't mean that stress is necessarily causing all of your symptoms; but it's a pretty good bet that if you're under a lot of stress, this has something to do with it. And if you reduce your stress, you might find that you have fewer medical complaints. Next, let's explore how stress can cause these physical symptoms.

Effects on Your Immune System

Have you had a cold lately? How did you catch it? Were you around other people who had colds? Did someone sneeze on you? To catch a cold you first have to be exposed to the cold virus. But once you're exposed your level of stress plays a huge role in how severe your cold becomes, how long it lasts, and—believe it or not—whether you even get sick in the first place. In a fascinating set of studies, researchers exposed participants to cold viruses and then followed them closely for several weeks. They found that not only does the chance of getting sick increase when you have more stress, but the degree of stress is related to the length and severity (as measured by mucous levels) of your cold. Studies also show that certain stressful times of the year have high rates of illness. For example, on college campuses, the incidence of upper respiratory infections tends to increase around final exam time.

What exactly does stress have to do with colds and infections? What role does it play in making you sick? Simply put, stress weakens your body's *immune system*—the complex network of special cells, tissues, and organs that protects you from foreign materials called *antigens*. Antigens are like uninvited guests that enter your body in one way or another. Common antigens are things like bacteria, viruses, dust particles, and parasites. Because antigens are all around us, our immune system is constantly seeking them out. When it finds them, it produces antibodies, which literally surround the antigen and neutralize it. The immune system also "remembers" each different antigen, so if it is found again in your body, it is detected and neutralized quickly to keep you from getting sick.

But when you're stressed, levels of the hormone *cortisol* increase in your body, as mentioned in Chapter 1. While cortisol is helpful to the immune system in small quantities, constant stress floods the body with too much cortisol, which causes the immune system to stop functioning properly. As a result, your body becomes more susceptible to invading antigens that it cannot fight off or neutralize as easily. This translates to longer and more severe infections, colds, and other ailments. It might even take your body longer to recover from cuts, sores, and other minor injuries.

Stress and Pain

Lots of things can cause pain, but studies show that people who have greater stress tend to have more problems with headaches, lower back pain, and pain in the neck, shoulder, face, jaw, and joints. Why? It's simple. Stress causes muscle tension, and when your muscles are constantly tense, they become tired and fatigued. This is what leads to pain.

Your shoulders, neck, and back are particularly prone to stress-related pain because they hold you up and support your 10-pound head. Pain may start with bad habits like clenching your teeth or poor posture, but tension in neck and shoulder muscles makes the problem worse, often causing pain to radiate. Pain on the side of the face that can radiate to the head or neck may indicate a jaw problem known as temporomandibular joint (TMJ) disorder. But it's usually not the joint that's the real problem. It's the muscle tension from clenching your teeth while under stress.

The same kind of muscle tension also leads to tension headaches. And if you have frequent headaches, it puts you at higher risk for developing problems with depression and anxiety—in other words, more stress. So, the relationship between stress and pain is like a vicious cycle. Stress leads to pain and pain leads to more stress—and on and on it goes. If you have chronic problems with headaches, you might also consult your doctor to make sure nothing else is going on.

Cardiovascular Problems

Your heart, lungs, and blood vessels make up your cardiovascular system, and it, too, can be affected by chronic stress. For one thing, the stress response makes your heart work overtime, putting it under intense strain—the kind of serious strain that over months and years can lead this vital organ to weaken and stop working properly. As we'll see later in this chapter, stress is also associated with unhealthy behaviors such as smoking, drug and alcohol abuse, and poor eating habits, which also have harmful effects on your heart and lungs and can lead to clogged blood vessels. This increases your risk of serious conditions such as a heart attack, lung or liver disease, or stroke.

Stress and Asthma

Asthma is a chronic disease that causes "asthma attacks," in which breathing becomes difficult and the person wheezes, coughs, and feels tightness in the chest. During attacks, the airways in your lungs become inflamed and narrowed, the muscles that surround these airways tighten, and the airways fill up with mucus. This is a bad combination! For some people, asthma is nothing more than a nuisance; but for others it can be a matter of life and death. And although stress doesn't cause you to get asthma in the first place, if you happen to have it, it does affect how often you have attacks and how severe the attacks are. How does this work? Since stress weakens the immune system, antigens, irritants, and infections (such as pollen, mold, pet dander, certain foods, cigarette smoke, cold and flu viruses) have a clearer path to your lungs, where they cause irritation that leads to asthma attacks.

Irritable Bowel Syndrome (IBS)

IBS is a digestive system disorder that causes stomach pain, constipation, diarrhea, bloating, or gas, and abdominal cramps. For some people, IBS is a minor condition; but for others, it's chronic, painful, and embarrassing. While the exact cause of IBS is unknown, it's clear that (once again) stress can make the symptoms worse. This occurs because the hormones released during the stress response (namely, cortisol and adrenaline) affect the nerve endings in your gut, causing all sorts of upheaval with your digestive system, such as increased mucous secretions, changes in the speed and strength of the contractions in your colon, and the experience of stomach pain.

Stress and Hair Loss

Excessive stress can even cause hair loss. Your hair might temporarily stop growing and fall out, but then grow back within several months. In more severe cases, hair follicles all over your body might die and treatment might be required to allow the hair to grow back.

HOW IS STRESS AFFECTING YOUR MIND?

Do these scenarios sound familiar?

- You're late for an important dinner meeting, there's no sign of the babysitter, the dog needs to be walked, and your toddler is about to stick a screwdriver in the electrical outlet. You go to shout at her to stop, but you come up empty—or you call her by her brother's name!

- It's final exam time—you've got to do well to keep your grade point average up. After studying all day, you decide to take a study break to get some food. You need some cash, so you go to the ATM on campus. A few hours later you realize that you left your ATM card in the machine.

Do situations like these mean you're totally losing it? Not really. But the very high levels of adrenaline and cortisol released during prolonged stress can actually curb your thinking processes and derail your ability to recall information that you clearly know. Stress can make you feel (and act) "scattered" and unable to think carefully or focus on a conversation or task. Chronic stress, in fact, may actually damage brain cells.

The following checklist contains 25 mental symptoms that can be related to stress. Put a check mark next to any that you've experienced over the past month. Then put the total number of symptoms you've experienced in the blank at the bottom of the checklist.

❒ Forgetfulness

❒ Trouble remembering familiar things (names of your children, objects)

❒ Trouble concentrating at work/school

❒ Letting minor things "get to you"

❒ Constant worrying

❒ Thoughts of death

❒ Trouble making decisions (even easy ones)

❒ Feeling hopeless

❒ Feeling like your day should be more productive

❒ Feeling distracted

❒ Constantly thinking the worst (jumping to conclusions)

❒ Feeling helpless

❒ Blowing things out of proportion

❒ Trouble looking at the "bright side" of things

❒ Becoming preoccupied with your problems

❒ Feeling rejected

❒ Trouble being able to laugh

❒ Worrying about having too much free time

❑ Feeling like you can't talk to others about your problems

❑ Feeling like you're always under pressure

❑ Feeling like you haven't accomplished enough

❑ Trouble being patient with others

❑ Feeling like other people are always wrong

❑ Feeling reluctant to take a vacation

❑ Dreading the weekends

_____ **Total number of symptoms**

What was your score (how many items did you check)? Research shows that people who experience higher levels of stress tend to experience more of these problems. As with the physical symptoms, stress may not necessarily be the cause of all of these, but rest assured that it's not helping you, and is most likely making things worse. Here again, reducing your stress can improve these mental processes.

How does stress influence your thinking? In Chapter 1 you learned about the mental part of the fight-or-flight response. Under the direction of adrenaline and cortisol, certain parts of your brain automatically spring to action during stress. Stress leads to an increase in alertness and attention. But it's not the good kind of alertness and attention. Instead, your mind automatically gets locked into thinking about the source of the stress. You become preoccupied—unable to take your mind off your troubles. That's why if you're with other people, they might notice that you seem like you're lost in thought, distant, or not paying attention. The fact is that you *are* paying attention—very close attention—but *only* to what's got you so stressed out. Talk about a one-track mind!

If you think about it, this is actually a useful effect of the fight-or-flight response. After all, if something inside didn't automatically shift our attention (and lock it) to things that could be harmful or threatening to us, we might not survive. But too much of this has the opposite effect: your mind has only so many resources; and when most of them are focused on the stressor, there's not much left to go around. The result? Your mind becomes fatigued and you have trouble concentrating on everyday activities; you forget people's names; you have trouble remembering simple routines; you focus on the worst possible outcome; and your judgment even becomes impaired. Research shows that long-term stress can even *permanently* harm your brain functioning: in one study, people exposed to high stress for just 3 to 6 years showed impaired memory and learning skills.

HOW IS STRESS AFFECTING YOUR FEELINGS AND EMOTIONS?

Does it seem like you're on an emotional roller coaster these days? Are you getting angry more often? Do you have crying spells? Do you have trouble relaxing? Everyone's emotional response to stress differs. And different stressors may bring out different emotions in you. Work- or school-related stress may result in anxiety. An argument with a friend, spouse, or partner might lead to anger and frustration. An accumulation of daily hassles might provoke irritability and moodiness. The loss of an important relationship or the death of a loved one might provoke feelings of depression.

Things had been going great for Roy, a high-level manager of a large bank, until his new boss, Sandy, began piling on the work. Roy would get phone calls and e-mails from Sandy demanding that work be done immediately—even when they had agreed to a later deadline. Sandy never gave praise for good work, only negative feedback if things weren't exactly as she expected. Within a few weeks, Roy was having daily crying spells. He would wake up in the middle of the night with anxiety attacks. He had to take a leave of absence to deal with all of his stress.

Amy was having a terrible week. On Monday, the car broke down and she had to spend all day at the dealership waiting for it to be repaired. She had to miss her long-awaited tennis game with her friends. On Tuesday, her toddler came down with a cold. Wednesday brought news that someone had stolen her husband's credit card and made lots of expensive purchases. On Thursday, her son was sent to the school principal's office for fighting and Amy had to pick him up early. By Friday, Amy was very moody and irritable. Every little thing seemed to set her off. She even lashed out verbally at her husband when he asked her if she had seen his car keys.

Core Beliefs Linked to Stressful Emotions

Feeling/emotion	Type of core belief	Examples
Depression	Incompetent	"I'm a failure"; "I'm not good enough"; "I'm stupid."
Depression	Unlovable/worthless	"I'm worthless"; "I don't matter"; "I'm bad/defective."
Guilt	Demanding (of yourself)	"I should be perfect"; "I must always please everyone."
Anger	Demanding (of others)	"People should behave the right way"; "Others must follow the rules."
Anxiety	Helpless	"I am weak"; "I can't cope"; "The world is a dangerous place"; "People are out to get me."
Anger/anxiety	Perfectionistic	"I must have control over things."
Anger/anxiety	Awfulizing/catastrophizing	"It's horrible when things don't go the way I want them to"; "I can't stand it when something goes wrong."

The checklist below contains some of the major emotional symptoms often associated with stress. Check the boxes next to any that you've experienced over the past few months. Then add up the number of checks you made and write the total in the blank that appears after the checklist.

❑ Crying spells

❑ A short temper

❑ Trouble relaxing

❑ Feeling agitated

❑ Feeling keyed up or on edge

❑ Anxiety

❑ Feeling insecure

❑ Depression and unhappiness

❑ A sense of loneliness

❑ Being easily startled

❑ Feeling overwhelmed

❑ Worrying

❑ Feeling socially isolated

_____ **Total number of symptoms**

How many boxes did you check? Although other things could explain why you have these symptoms, it's likely that stress plays a role, too. Later in this chapter, you'll examine whether your problems with stress rise to the level of a clinical anxiety or mood *disorder*—psychological problems that usually require immediate professional help.

How does stress influence your emotions and feelings? It's simple: *by influencing how you think*. It's a fact that how you feel depends on your basic assumptions and attitudes about yourself, other people, and the world around you. Pioneering psychologists such as Albert Ellis and Aaron Beck observed that certain types of assumptions or "core beliefs" lead to certain emotions. You can think of core beliefs as part of your mental road map for how to live your life. Like voices in your mind, core beliefs help you make sense of the world. They help you develop a set of "rules" for how you should feel about certain situations. But people who have problems with stress tend to have maladaptive core beliefs, which trigger negative feelings and emotions. Check out the table on the previous page. It shows different types of negative core beliefs that produce the kinds of negative feelings and emotions that are associated with stress.

Like a sleeping giant, your maladaptive core beliefs might lie dormant most of the time, only to be roused and set in motion when under stress (remember that stress influences our thinking processes). In Chapter 8, you'll learn strategies for identifying, challenging, and revamping your maladaptive negative core beliefs into more helpful attitudes (it turns out this is one of the best ways to manage stress). For now, what's important is that you understand that stress affects your feelings and emotions by activating your negative core beliefs. Your core beliefs influence how you feel—and what you *do*, as we'll see next.

HOW IS STRESS AFFECTING YOUR BEHAVIOR?

Can you identify with these situations?

- It's 11:00 P.M. The day is over. The kids are in bed. But your mind is still going full tilt. You toss and turn in bed for what seems like hours.

- Not long ago, you finished a large meal. But now you find yourself aimlessly looking through the fridge or the pantry. You're probably not really hungry—just craving something to eat. But before you know it, you've binged on a plethora of unhealthy foods.

- Everyone is excited about the vacation—except *you*. You can't stop thinking that you've got too much work to do to enjoy a few days of rest and relaxation.

- You have trouble sitting still, foot tapping, pacing, nail biting, constantly shifting in your seat, or fidgeting with one thing or another.

Make no mistake about it; stress has detrimental effects on your behavior. It can lead to impulsiveness (acting without thinking carefully), unhealthy habits, treating others poorly, becoming socially isolated, and overworking yourself until you're literally exhausted. How has stress affected your behavior? Following are five categories of common problem behaviors related to too much stress. Mark the box next to any that you've noticed.

Quick fixes

❏ Smoking

❏ Increased alcohol use

❏ Increased drug use

❏ Overeating

❏ Excessive gambling or impulse buying

Pushing yourself too hard

☐ Pulling all-nighters

☐ "Overstudying" or "overpreparing"

☐ Trouble finding time to enjoy yourself

☐ Burnout (feeling totally overwhelmed and exhausted)

Antisocial/aggressive behavior

☐ Anger and hostility

☐ Extreme competitiveness

☐ Being sarcastic to others

☐ Relationship conflicts

☐ Destroying property when angry

☐ Not wanting to socialize (isolating yourself)

☐ Spending too much time talking about your problems

Using poor judgment

☐ Fast driving

☐ Engaging in other risky behaviors

☐ Having lots of accidents

Direct effects of stress

☐ Eating too little

☐ Reduced interest in sex

☐ Having trouble sitting (or standing) still

☐ Reduced work or school productivity

☐ Talking fast, sometimes leading to stuttering

☐ Trouble sleeping (insomnia)

☐ Excessive nail biting or skin picking

☐ Pulling out hairs from your head or other parts of your body

☐ Pacing, foot tapping, nervous laughter

_____ **Total number of symptoms**

How many boxes did you check, and from which categories? Let's learn about how stress causes these different types of behaviors—and how these behaviors can actually create more stress.

Quick Fixes

Most people have healthy and adaptive ways of coping with stress, for example, venting or problem solving with friends or family. Others hit the gym and lift weights or take to the streets and go running. Some people meditate or pray; others lose themselves in their favorite video game, TV show, or movie. Musicians might turn to their instrument, and painters to their canvas, in stressful times. But some stress-related behaviors are maladaptive or dangerous—especially those that involve the use of substances that create an artificial feeling of well-being. Cigarette smoking is the perfect example of such a "quick fix." The nicotine in cigarettes causes the brain to release chemicals, such as endorphins, that actually raise your mood for a while. Lighting up and smoking also distracts you from thinking about or dealing with stressors, and because it's often a social activity, you might associate smoking with positive feelings of comfort and support. It's no wonder research shows that people with high levels of stress are twice as likely to be smokers as those who are less stressed.

Alcohol and many types of drugs are also maladaptive quick fixes for stress because they artificially produce a mindset of relaxation or pleasure. Where stress increases alertness and anxiety, alcohol and many other drugs diminish these feelings, leaving you less worried about the situation. They create a diversion from healthy coping and hinder your ability to address the real problem; so when their effects wear off, you're right back where you started. And if the stressful situation continues for a long time, it can lead to substance *abuse* and becoming *dependent*. It's a vicious cycle: using alcohol and drugs to escape from stressful feelings, which prevents healthy coping and prolongs stressors turning to substances again and again, causing further delay in healthy coping. Fill out the Eye Opener on the facing page to see if you might need help dealing with substance use.

Similarly, eating is a pleasurable behavior that can temporarily reduce stress (this is called "emotional eating"). Perhaps you have particular "comfort foods" that you turn to when feeling stressed. Foods that are high in fat, salt, and carbohydrates make us feel better because they taste good and produce changes in the brain that cause a temporary feeling of well-being. You're especially likely to overeat if you're under constant stress because the prolonged release of adrenaline and cortisol causes hunger and sets off food cravings. These chemicals also make your body store fat, increasing the chances that you'll pack on the pounds.

Excessive gambling and impulse buying (that is, making large purchases just to help yourself feel better) are also often used as stress relievers and diversions. But these behaviors don't actually help you solve the real problems in your life, and in fact, might create new ones (for example, financial strain).

EYE OPENER

Do You Suffer from a Substance Use Disorder?

You're not alone if you do. Many people with stress misuse drugs and alcohol to the point that it interferes with their lives. Here's a list of the symptoms. If your frequent use of drugs or alcohol has resulted in any of the following, it's worth seeking professional help:

❐ Problems with work (for example, poor job performance), school (for example, repeated absences or suspensions), or at home (such as neglecting children or important household tasks).

❐ Legal problems (such as arrests) for substance-related disorderly conduct.

❐ Substance use in potentially dangerous situations (such as driving or operating a machine when intoxicated).

❐ Frequent social or interpersonal problems (such as physical fights or arguments with your spouse about too much drug use).

Pushing Yourself Too Hard

If work, school, or projects around the house are a source of stress for you, it might seem like the obvious thing to do is just work harder.

- You stay up all night to study for the big exam.

- You work on the weekends instead of taking a break to enjoy yourself.

- You avoid socializing and other pleasurable activities as if you have to punish yourself for not working hard enough or achieving enough.

- You push yourself so hard that you find yourself losing interest in whatever it is you're doing.

These maladaptive behaviors result from rigid core beliefs (as described earlier) such as "Anything less than perfection isn't good enough" or "I don't deserve to enjoy myself." These are maladaptive because they consistently lead you to push yourself too hard. But the ironic thing is that pushing yourself to the limit—and beyond—can lead to *burnout*, in which your performance suffers, you lose motivation, get down on yourself . . . and you're right back where you started.

When you constantly push yourself to be absolutely perfect all the time, you raise your stress level to the point that it actually keeps you from doing your best.

Antisocial/Aggressive Behavior

The tendency to be aggressive, competitive, or hostile when you're under stress is difficult to resist. It's the *fight* part of the fight-or-flight response, and therefore normal. But if your fuse is really short and you don't have skills for managing anger and frustration, it might lead to outbursts of physical or verbal aggression. You might be easily irritated, leading you to become hostile to those around you or lose control and destroy things, perhaps creating tension in your relationships. Most of the time, this type of behavior only compounds your stress level.

Maybe, like some people, you retreat from others when you feel stressed. Instead of seeking advice or comfort from those around you, you isolate yourself. Some people seek out others, but then can't seem to talk about anything but their own stressful situations. Although it's natural to be preoccupied with thinking about stressors, it's poor social skills to dwell on your problems and perseverate about them with other people.

Using Poor Judgment

Because stress impairs your ability to make thoughtful decisions, you might be prone to engaging in risky behaviors that put you or others in harm's way. Speeding, driving under the influence of drugs or alcohol, and picking fights are some examples. But you might generally be more likely to take risks, more prone to rush through things, and less careful. Do you have more accidents, mishaps, and collisions, or make more mistakes than you should? Stress might be to blame.

Direct Effects of Stress

Since stress is associated with a general increase in physical arousal, it's common to feel keyed up, on edge, and on the go when you're on stress overload. This will cause you to have trouble sleeping, concentrating, and even sitting still. Sleep loss is a particularly serious problem because when you're sleep deprived, your threshold for dealing with stressors is even lower—keeping you stressed out and making it more difficult to sleep the following night.

If you can't actually fight or flee from your stressors, the nervous energy created by the stress response may manifest itself in other ways, such as nervous habits. Nail biting, skin picking, hair pulling, talking rapidly (sometimes stuttering), pacing, foot or finger tapping, and nervous laughter are common examples. While some people overeat in response to stress (as described earlier), others lose their appetite, eat too little, and lose dangerous amounts of weight or deplete important bodily nutrients. You might also experience a reduction in your sex drive, induced by the continued release of stress hormones.

IS IT STRESS OR AN ANXIETY DISORDER?

Stress and anxiety have many similarities. Both involve the fight-or-flight response, and both lead to many of the problems discussed in this chapter (such as loss of sleep, maladaptive behavior, and feelings of depression). But whereas stress is a normal reaction designed to help you adapt to situations that are unexpected or that take you out of your usual routine, *anxiety* is an intense feeling of apprehension or fear. *Anxiety disorders* are a group of psychological problems characterized by excessive or unreasonable fear and apprehension that typically require professional help. People with these problems have symptoms every day that cause intense distress and interfere with daily activities and relationships. The strategies in this workbook are very effective in helping people reduce their daily stress levels. But if you suffer from one or more of the following anxiety disorders, you might require professional help.

Generalized Anxiety Disorder

This is a problem characterized by excessive and uncontrollable worrying. You spend more than half the day (50% of your waking hours) worrying unnecessarily about things like your own and others' health, family issues or other relationships, finances, the future, your job, or your studies. The worry becomes so severe that it gets in the way of your work or school performance and prevents you from enjoying your free time. It also leads to physical problems such as low energy, aching, sore muscles, and exhaustion. You might feel antsy during the day and then have difficulty sleeping at night. Emotionally, you might feel testy, snapping at people and easily aggravated.

Panic Attacks

These are recurring (sometimes unexpected) episodes of intense fear that start abruptly and reach a peak within a few minutes. They might involve feeling like something awful is about to happen to you (like a feeling of intense dread) or the urge to run away from the situation you're in. Some people say they feel like they're losing their mind or about to lose their self-control. Racing or pounding heart, trouble catching your breath, perspiring, shaking, or dizziness may make you feel as if you're about to have a heart attack. Panic can feel so uncomfortable and frightening that people often start to avoid the people, events, or situations that they associate with having an attack, which can make leading a normal life challenging.

Obsessive–Compulsive Disorder (OCD)

OCD involves two types of symptoms: One type, *obsessions*, consists of uninvited, unwelcome, upsetting thoughts that come up over and over, despite the fact that they seem to make no sense. Examples of obsessions include an irrational fear of contracting an infection or a disease from normal activities like using the washroom, fear that you'll leave the windows or doors unlocked and someone will break into your house, or the belief that you have harmed or will harm someone through a violent act. Sometimes obsessions take shape as detailed thoughts; other times they are just images, like pictures that flash in your mind. The anxiety and fear that you feel may not be specific but rather just an overwhelming dread that if things aren't "just right"—even, lined up, balanced, or a certain number, for example—something terrible will happen. The other symptom is *compulsions*, urges to go through certain prescribed mental or behavioral routines or rituals, such as excessive washing/cleaning (if you were afraid of getting sick), checking (such as the windows and doors), repeating everyday behaviors (like tying your shoes), counting, arranging/ordering (lining up the coffee cups "perfectly" in your kitchen cabinet, for example), and asking for assurances that your obsession will not come true. While most everyone experiences obsessions and compulsions from time to time, people with full-blown OCD have these symptoms for hours each day and to the point that they interfere with the daily routine. The symptoms of OCD often get worse or extend to new obsessions and compulsions over time.

Phobias

A phobia is an extreme and unjustified fear, which often feels like panic when it comes over you, of something specific, such as fear of flying, fear of heights, of certain animals (like dogs or bugs), of hypodermics, or of anything else. One separate, broader type of phobia, called *social phobia*, involves fear of social situations, from conversations to parties to meetings. Most people who suffer from phobias go to great lengths to avoid what they are afraid of, which, as with OCD, can impose severe limits on their daily lives, depending on their specific phobia.

Anxiety disorders have some overlapping features with stress—physical reactions, maladaptive thinking patterns, maladaptive behaviors—but professional help is usually required to reduce the extreme fear and apprehension and the avoidance patterns. If you have the symptoms of an anxiety disorder, it is worth consulting with a psychologist or psychiatrist. The good news is that these problems are usually treatable with CBT.

WHAT COULD STRESS DO TO YOU IF YOU DON'T HELP YOURSELF?

So, now that you know the ins and outs of how stress works, and the different ways it might be affecting you in the near term, let's examine what's at stake in the long run—that is, what can happen to you if you don't *address your stress*.

EYE PENER

Getting Help for an Anxiety Disorder

Anxiety disorders are the most common mental health problems. But they're also among the most treatable. The best form of treatment is cognitive-behavioral therapy (CBT), which involves learning and practicing skills for changing the thinking and behavioral patterns that are present with severe anxiety. For more information (including listings of places to turn for help), visit the Anxiety and Depression Association of America's website at *www.adaa.org*.

With the experience of continuous or repetitive stress over the years, the levels of cortisol and adrenaline in your bloodstream stay high and the impairments in physical, cognitive, emotional, and behavioral functioning become more and more pronounced. The body begins to experience each stressor as an extra burden due to the side effects of the persistently high stress hormones, and irreversible physical damage to the brain and other vital organs (such as the heart and digestive system) sets in. The manifestations could be devastating.

Cardiovascular Disease

Over the long term, people with higher stress levels have a higher risk of cardiovascular diseases such as heart attacks, coronary artery disease, and strokes. This risk is particularly high if you tend to be excessively competitive, impatient, and hostile, and move and talk quickly (sometimes called "Type A Personality"). Research shows that of these characteristics, hostility is the most significant predictor of developing heart disease. The common stress response of eating comfort foods, with their accompanying fat and salt, further increases the risk.

Hypertension (high blood pressure) is a common condition that can be deadly if undetected. If you have a family history of hypertension and heart problems, it's a good idea to have regular checkups with your doctor.

High Blood Pressure

Also known as *hypertension*, this is a chronic disease that usually has no obvious symptoms. But it raises your risk of stroke, heart failure, kidney failure, and heart attacks. Recall that the release of adrenaline during stressful periods raises your blood pressure. It does so by narrowing your blood vessels (by causing blood vessel walls to constrict). So, frequently repeated or prolonged stress can lead to a permanent state of high blood pressure.

Hypertension is very common in modern society and presents a serious medical problem because it is directly related to strokes, heart disease, arteriosclerosis (hardening of the arteries), and kidney failure.

Susceptibility to Infection

You've already read how chronic stress suppresses the immune system, making you more vulnerable to infections. Allergies, asthma, and autoimmune diseases (including arthritis and multiple sclerosis) may be exacerbated by stress. If you're under lots of stress, the rate at which you recover from any illnesses will be slowed.

Skin Problems

Acne, psoriasis, and eczema, which are themselves very stressful, have also been linked to constant, long-term stress.

If you're thinking that stress is a dire problem, you're right. It is. But the good news is that if you act now, you can avoid its long-term ill effects. And you've already completed an important step: After reading Chapters 1 and 2, you're now an expert on the inner workings of stress. In Chapters 3 and 4 I'll help you identify the particular stressors in your life (Chapter 3) and design a plan for what you can do about them (Chapter 4).

EYE PENER

The Link between Stress and Medical Problems

The connection between your health and your stress level is undeniable. Take air traffic controllers, for example. They have one of the most stressful jobs possible, with continual responsibility for the lives of thousands of people. Unfortunately, people who work in this job are also five times more likely than the rest of us to suffer from high blood pressure (hypertension).

3

What's Stressing You Out?

At first, the answer to the question posed in the title of this chapter might seem straightforward—but it's not that simple. That's because stress actually comes from three types of sources: (1) *events and situations* (including those that involve other people), (2) *thoughts* (your ideas, perceptions, and beliefs), and (3) *negative emotions* (such as anxiety, anger, and depression). And to complicate things further, these sources of stress are linked together. So, to manage stress effectively, you'll need to understand your own situational triggers, stress-provoking thinking patterns, and stress-inducing emotional states. In this chapter you'll learn the connections among situations, thoughts, and emotions, and I'll help you pinpoint those that stress you out.

SITUATIONS, THOUGHTS, AND FEELINGS: HOW ARE THEY RELATED?

It's easy to think that everyone experiences stress in a similar way. Wouldn't anyone be stressed out by an unexpected job loss? Doesn't everyone lose sleep at night worrying about a child whose grades have plummeted? Not necessarily. For a long time, experts believed that the same stressful event (stressor) would cause everyone to become about equally stressed. After lots of research, though, we know that's not true. The truth is that events and situations are not entirely to blame for feelings of stress. Everyone experiences most situations and events differently. As a matter of fact, two people can be in the same negative circumstance, but their individual stress levels may be completely different. Consider the story of Jamie and Melissa and their canceled flight:

Jamie and Melissa are best friends, and they're getting ready to go on vacation together. They're at the airport waiting for their flight, but it's snowing heavily and they've just learned that all flights to their destination have been canceled for the day. Jamie takes this very hard. She is thinking, "This is awful. We'll never get there. Our vacation is ruined. I always get all the bad luck. It's so unfair." Melissa looks at the situation differently. To her, it's more of a nuisance than a catastrophe. She says to herself, "I wish this wasn't happening, but you can't control the weather. I guess we'll have to make the best of it—there really isn't anything else we can do at this point. This will be an experience we'll never forget."

It might not surprise you to learn that Jamie was much more stressed out about the canceled flight than Melissa. Jamie grew more and more irritable, losing her cool and even snapping at the ticket agent who was trying to help them get booked on a flight the next day. She felt helpless and sick to her stomach, and developed a headache. Melissa, on the other hand, while disappointed and frustrated, remained composed and cooperative. She didn't have the strong negative feelings or physical symptoms that her friend Jamie was having. She coped much better with the stressful situation.

How can two friends in the same situation have such different stress levels? The answer has to do with how we *think about* the situation. Jamie viewed the canceled flight as a *total catastrophe*. She blew it out of proportion ("The vacation is ruined") and took it personally ("I always get all the bad luck"). This type of thinking led to Jamie's feeling helpless, depressed, angry, and anxious. And these intense negative emotions made her lose her cool and become uncooperative. Melissa, on the other hand, was thinking more rationally. She didn't like the situation, but she also realized that there wasn't much she could do about it, so she'd have to cope the best she could. This kind of thinking helped Melissa keep her stress levels in check.

THE ABC'S OF STRESS

The moral of Jamie and Melissa's story is that while events and situations influence your stress level to some degree, *how you think about these events* has even more to do with how stressed out you become. That's because your thinking patterns intensify your emotional response to the stressor. And intense feelings of anger, helplessness, anxiety, and depression impair your ability to cope with the stressor, making the situation even worse and creating a vicious cycle. Psychologist Albert Ellis referred to this cycle using an ABC model in which "A" is the stressful event that *activates* the cycle, "B" is the thinking pattern or *belief system* that intensifies negative emotions about "A," and "C" represents the emotional and behavioral *consequences* of the thoughts and beliefs. The diagram below

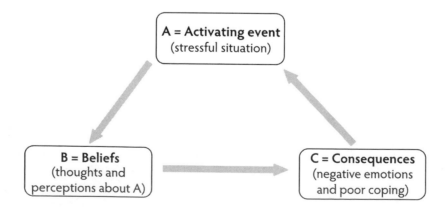

shows how activating events (A's), beliefs (B's), and emotional/behavioral consequences (C's) are related in a vicious cycle.

Next, let's identify the A's, B's, and C's in your life that cause you stress. We'll start with the A's.

IDENTIFYING YOUR A's: STRESSFUL EVENTS

Because the A's are what set the wheels of stress in motion, becoming aware of them will help you get the most out of the strategies in this workbook. Think about the past year. What were the big changes in your life? What about the ongoing challenges that you've had to cope with? The list of 43 events and circumstances on page 46–47 was developed by psychiatrists Thomas Holmes and Richard Rahe. They found that these were the events most associated with stress. As you read through the list, consider whether any have happened to you in the last year. If so, place a check in the box next to the event. Then write a brief description of the event in the right-hand column.

In addition to these "big-ticket" life events, stress can be triggered by less severe *daily hassles*—traffic, a crying baby, waiting in line, bad weather, and other aggravations. And research shows that the stress of dealing with these hassles one after another, day after day, actually causes the most stress-related health problems. The list on page 48–49 includes common daily hassles that people report as being stressful. As with the previous list, check the box next to any hassles that have been hampering you recently. Use the right-hand column to write a description of the hassle and how it affects you.

Did I miss anything? In the following blanks, write in any additional significant life events or hassles that you didn't see mentioned in the lists that trigger stress.

_____

_____

_____

_____

If you're stressed out by one or more of the life events or hassles in the two lists that you just read, an obvious way to reduce your stress is to change the situation or avoid it altogether. Having trouble with office politics? Just stay out of it. Does the cold or rainy weather where you live stress you out? Move to a warmer, drier climate. Don't like flying in airplanes? Drive or keep travel to a minimum. To a certain extent, stress management is about problem solving and developing a plan for changing the situations and circumstances that trigger stress. You'll learn some ways of doing this in Part II of this book.

But this approach will get you only so far. What if you can't change the situation? What if you can't avoid the stressor? You get pulled into office politics without realizing

TYPICALLY STRESSFUL EVENTS

Event or circumstance	Description
☐ 1. Death of a spouse	
☐ 2. Divorce	
☐ 3. Marital separation	
☐ 4. Jail term	
☐ 5. Death of a close family member	
☐ 6. Personal injury or illness	
☐ 7. Marriage	
☐ 8. Fired from work	
☐ 9. Marital reconciliation	
☐ 10. Retirement	
☐ 11. Change in health of family member	
☐ 12. Pregnancy or new baby	
☐ 13. Sex difficulties	
☐ 14. Poverty	
☐ 15. Being in debt	
☐ 16. Change in financial state	
☐ 17. Death of close friend	
☐ 18. Change to a different line of work	
☐ 19. Frequent arguments with spouse or partner	
☐ 20. Mortgage over $10,000	
☐ 21. Foreclosure of mortgage or loan	

Adapted with permission from Holmes, T. H., and Rahe, R. H. (1967). The second readjustment rating scale. *Journal of Psychosomatic Research*, *11*, 213–218. Copyright 1967 by Elsevier Limited.

Event or circumstance	Description
☐ 22. Change in responsibilities at work	
☐ 23. Child leaving home	
☐ 24. Trouble with in-laws	
☐ 25. Outstanding personal achievement	
☐ 26. Spouse begins or stops work	
☐ 27. Begin or end school	
☐ 28. Change in living conditions	
☐ 29. Business readjustment	
☐ 30. Trouble with boss	
☐ 31. Change in work hours or conditions	
☐ 32. Change in residence	
☐ 33. Change in schools	
☐ 34. Change in recreational activities	
☐ 35. Change in religious affiliation or place of worship	
☐ 36. Change in social activities	
☐ 37. Mortgage or loan less than $10,000	
☐ 38. Change in sleeping habits or sleep schedule	
☐ 39. Change in number of family get-togethers	
☐ 40. Change in eating habits	
☐ 41. Vacation	
☐ 42. Major holiday get-together (such as Thanksgiving or Christmas)	
☐ 43. Minor violations of the law	

TYPICALLY STRESSFUL DAILY HASSLES

Daily hassle	Description
❑ 1. Excess noise (crying babies, car horns, etc.)	
❑ 2. Bureaucracy or office politics	
❑ 3. Misplaced or lost items (keys, phone, etc.)	
❑ 4. Arguments	
❑ 5. Waiting in lines	
❑ 6. Inconsiderate people	
❑ 7. Difficult neighbors	
❑ 8. Loneliness	
❑ 9. Traffic jams	
❑ 10. Time pressures	
❑ 11. Car troubles	
❑ 12. Deadlines at work or school	
❑ 13. Concerns about crime	
❑ 14. Shopping	
❑ 15. Large crowds	

Daily hassle	Description
☐ 16. Pollution	
☐ 17. Relatives	
☐ 18. Gossip	
☐ 19. Cooking/food preparation	
☐ 20. Frequent traveling (such as driving long distances, flying, a long commute to work)	
☐ 21. Problems with children	
☐ 22. Exposure to negative news stories	
☐ 23. Political debates and controversies	
☐ 24. Harassment or bullying from others	
☐ 25. Colds and allergies	
☐ 26. Bad or extreme weather (such as snow, a cold snap, or a heat wave)	
☐ 27. Boredom	
☐ 28. Speaking in public or to a group of people	
☐ 29. Exams or job interviews	
☐ 30. Broken appliances (such as the computer, air conditioner, or refrigerator)	
☐ 31. House repairs	

it. You can't just relocate to a different climate because of where your job and family are based. You have important business trips and can't avoid flying. And many significant life events are beyond our control—major illness, a death in the family, your mother-in-law's behavior. When you can't control stressful situations themselves (or the people who create them), you'll need to focus on the B's—that is, you'll need to control how you *think* about them.

IDENTIFYING YOUR B's: STRESS-INDUCING BELIEFS AND THOUGHTS

Although stressful situations (A's) are often beyond your control, the good news is that your thoughts and beliefs—your B's—are within your control. And since, as we've seen, B's play a huge role in problems with stress, a major part of stress management is learning to recognize and change the sorts of thinking patterns that intensify your emotions and lead to poor coping. We'll get to the particulars of how to *change* maladaptive B's in Chapter 8. For now, though, it's important to learn about the types of maladaptive thinking that create your stress.

We're constantly monitoring and judging the situations around us, deciding whether each is good or bad for us, safe or dangerous.

Like Jamie and Melissa (described earlier), we all have a belief system about how the world works, and we have internal dialogues in which we make judgments and comments to ourselves about what we experience. Our thoughts and beliefs are often automatic and instantaneous (in fact, psychologists call them "automatic thoughts"). You see someone you haven't seen in a long time and think to yourself, "Wow, she looks great!" As you scan a restaurant menu, you say to yourself, "I bet the pork tenderloin is good—but mmm, I can just taste the salmon." You might not even realize these thoughts are occurring. But even so, they play an important role in your problems with stress. Here's how.

Researchers have found that people who are highly stressed have particular patterns of beliefs and automatic thoughts that are inaccurate or that exaggerate and distort their perception of reality. In general, they believe that the world is full of negatives and that they don't have as much control over these negatives as they should. It's this belief system that intensifies stress in stressful situations. Think about Jamie. As if having her flight canceled wasn't stressful enough, she made herself more stressed with catastrophic thinking that magnified her feelings of helplessness. The stress-related thinking patterns listed in the box on the facing page come from the work of Albert Ellis, as well as psychiatrists David Burns and Aaron Beck. You'll need to be able to recognize them if you're going to manage stress. In Chapter 8 you'll learn how to get out of these patterns as a technique for reducing your stress.

To help you identify the beliefs and attitudes that affect your stress levels, each of the following sections begins with three statements for you to consider. Decide whether you

---

Stress-Related Thinking Patterns

All-or-Nothing (Black-and-White) Thinking: You think in black-and-white terms—there are no in-betweens or shades of gray. A situation is either wonderful or awful.

Musturbation **("Must" and "Should" Statements):** You believe your happiness depends on things going as you think they *must* or *should* go. People *must* do as you wish. Things *should* turn out as you want.

Jumping to Conclusions: Even though it hasn't happened yet, you automatically assume that something dreadful is just around the corner.

Awfulizing and "What If?" Thinking: You imagine the worst possible (101% bad) outcome and then treat it as a foregone conclusion.

"I-Can't-Stand-Its" (Low Frustration Tolerance): You see yourself as unable to cope with a stressful situation.

Labeling: You attach an extreme negative label to yourself, someone else, or an event.

---

agree or disagree with each one and check the appropriate box. Then read more about each thinking pattern.

All-or-Nothing (Black-and-White) Thinking

I often see things as either *perfect* or *awful* with no middle ground. ❏ Agree ❏ Disagree

I frequently use terms like "always," "never," "everyone," and "no one." ❏ Agree ❏ Disagree

Something isn't worth doing if I can't do it perfectly. ❏ Agree ❏ Disagree

If you agreed with one or more of the preceding statements, you might have a habit of thinking in all-or-nothing terms—like a perfectionist. Your work is either absolutely *perfect* or a complete *failure*. Your child is either totally *brilliant* or utterly *stupid*. There are no shades of gray. No middle ground. This type of inflexible thinking often creates stress because in reality things are rarely all good or all bad—they're usually somewhere in the middle. And remember that we don't usually have complete control over these things anyway. So you're apt to find yourself angry, frustrated, and *stressed* over lots of things. For example, Carly worked as a camp counselor. At her evaluation, her supervisor said Carly was an excellent counselor in virtually every way but that she should work on being on time to staff meetings. Carly became very upset because her evaluation wasn't *perfect.* Of course, this was unrealistic. Carly could still be an excellent counselor without being 100% perfect.

Musturbation (Demandingness)

People should always treat me with kindness and respect.   ❏ Agree   ❏ Disagree

I must be successful, respected, and attractive, or else I can't be happy.   ❏ Agree   ❏ Disagree

Things should be comfortable and as I want them.   ❏ Agree   ❏ Disagree

Bill and a date were dining at an elegant restaurant. The place was jammed, and it took some extra time for the server to bring their food. Then Bill's salad arrived with dressing on it when Bill had specifically asked for it to be served on the side. Later the server brought dessert but forgot to offer coffee. Bill became livid—and stressed. His asthma even flared up. Sure, it was an inconvenience waiting a few extra minutes to be served, and it was a nuisance that he had to get another salad and remind the server about the coffee. But what really ramped up Bill's stress were his beliefs (B's) about the whole experience: "Fine restaurants *must* treat their customers with respect" and "I *should* have a competent waiter since I'm paying so much money for my food."

If you agreed with one or more of the statements in the preceding checklist, you— like Bill—probably have rules, standards, or *requirements* for how you think other people *should* behave or how things *must* go (*mus*turbation). And it's as if you can't be happy unless these standards are met. But we can't always control situations and people; and everyone makes mistakes. So, these sorts of unbending rules and demands are bound to be broken from time to time, leaving you angry, frustrated, and resentful, which adds to your stress. You might even use *shoulds* and *musts* to try to motivate yourself to be perfect. For example, "I *shouldn't* make mistakes" or "I *must* not let other people see my faults." It's like you can't be happy unless you're perfect. But is it really possible to be perfect all the time?

Jumping to Conclusions

If something can go wrong, it probably will.   ❏ Agree   ❏ Disagree

I seem to get all the bad luck.   ❏ Agree   ❏ Disagree

Even if they don't say so, I can tell when people don't like me.   ❏ Agree   ❏ Disagree

If you agreed with some of the preceding statements, you probably jump to negative conclusions even without having solid evidence. Maybe you act like a fortune-teller or psychic who believes he or she can see the future—but you mainly predict negative things for yourself. Then you assume your predictions are a proven fact, *before they even happen.* For example, "It just feels like I won't get the job" versus "I don't know if I'll get the job—there's always a chance." You might be so convinced that your prediction is the absolute truth that you selectively look for evidence to back it up, ignoring evidence to the contrary and raising your stress level.

Another type of jumping to conclusions is when you decide that you know what someone else is thinking (as if you could read the person's mind—in fact, we therapists call this *mind reading*). You might be so convinced that someone is reacting negatively to you that you don't even bother looking for proof. For example, at a work party your boss doesn't come over to talk to you, and you think, "She's avoiding me because I'm not getting the promotion." It's possible, however, that your boss was simply caught up in conversation with someone else and couldn't break away. Jumping to conclusions is like striking out in your mind before you've even come up to bat!

It's Fred's wedding day—stressful enough for anyone. But Fred has already decided that his wife's family won't like him. When his in-laws act sincerely and seem to welcome Fred into their family with open arms, he assumes he "knows" their true feelings. "They're only acting nice because my fiancée told them to. It probably won't last very long," he tells himself. As a result, Fred's stress level is even higher than it needs to be. Jumping to conclusions increases your anxiety, fear, and anticipation.

Awfulizing and "What If?" Thinking

I tend to expect the worst.	❐ Agree	❐ Disagree
It's important to always prepare for the worst possible outcome of a situation.	❐ Agree	❐ Disagree
Many things I worry about end up turning out far better than I thought they would.	❐ Agree	❐ Disagree

Let's face it, sometimes things go wrong. Very wrong. And whether it's your goof up, someone else's fault, bad timing, or bad luck, these situations are stressful enough. Awfulizing—telling yourself that a situation is (or will be) far worse than it really is (like *101% awful*)—is a sure way to increase that stress and anxiety and put you at an even greater disadvantage. Let's say you've made a mistake on an important project at work. You might think your boss will be so upset that he'll fire you on the spot, you'll never find another job, your family will disown you because you're a good-for-nothing, and you'll end up on the street, poor and lonely for the rest of your miserable life. Do you catch the thinking process here? You've gone from making a mistake (which all of us do from time to time) to being homeless! Of course, in reality this situation is likely to play out differently—and probably not as catastrophically. So, awfulizing occurs when we look to the future and anticipate that everything that could go wrong actually will (perhaps even worse than imaginable). Then, in our mind, we create a reality around those negative thoughts, not bothering to consider that maybe we're exaggerating things.

A good way to tell if you're awfulizing is by the presence of questions beginning with "*What if . . . ?*" "*What if* no one ever wants to be with me?"; "*What if* I have to live like this for the rest of my life?"; "*What if* the doctor can't cure me?"; "*What if* I flunk out of school?" These "What if?" questions usually amount to nothing except an overactive imagination . . . and intense stress.

"I-Can't-Stand-Its" (Low Frustration Tolerance)

I get annoyed easily over nuisances, inconveniences, and hassles.	❏ Agree	❏ Disagree
I am impatient and have trouble putting up with frustrations in the short term, even when there is something to gain in the long run.	❏ Agree	❏ Disagree
I often procrastinate—putting difficult or onerous activities off until some future time.	❏ Agree	❏ Disagree

If you agreed with one or more of the preceding statements, you might fall prey to "I can't stand it" thinking, which leads to difficulty putting up with the usual aggravations and inconveniences of life that most people deal with more gracefully. Another term for this is "low frustration tolerance" (or LFT), because you easily become annoyed or discouraged. Take Barry, for instance, who was learning how to play the guitar but couldn't quite get that chord on a new song he was trying to figure out. He thought to himself, "To hell with this—it's too damn hard! I can't stand it! I give up!" This led him to become impatient and unhinged. He couldn't deal with the fact that learning to play his new song would take lots of practice, so he furiously smashed his guitar.

If you have LFT, you might seek immediate gratification even it means missing out on something important in the long run. Maybe you procrastinate too much or find yourself champing at the bit impatiently when you have to wait or work for what you want. Perhaps you've had trouble working on overcoming a problem such as weight gain or alcohol/drug addiction because you think that you *couldn't stand* the immediate discomfort of doing so. Believing that you *can't stand* discomfort only leads to anger, frustration, impatience, irritability, and disruptive behavior—all of which add fuel to the fire of stress.

Labeling

Most people are either good or bad.	❏ Agree	❏ Disagree
People who make lots of mistakes are not as worthy as people who make fewer mistakes.	❏ Agree	❏ Disagree
I often judge people based on their actions.	❏ Agree	❏ Disagree

> *Everyone gets frustrated over certain things, but not everyone lets it get in the way of his or her mental or physical health or well-being.*

When you label, you take something you did—often a mistake—and turn it into a personal weakness. Instead of labeling what you *did* ("Boy, that was a stupid thing to do"), you mentally slap *yourself* with a negative label ("*I'm* stupid"). Often, the label is extreme: "I'm a *complete* loser" or worse. This sort of self-labeling leads to feelings of guilt and depression. So, if making a mistake or acting poorly doesn't cause you enough stress in the first place, beating yourself up this way is sure to send your stress levels that much higher.

You might also apply labeling to other people when their behavior bothers you. Someone cuts you off in traffic and you think, "What a jerk!" A coworker makes a mistake on a project and you tell yourself, "He's a fool!" Your husband is having trouble standing up to his boss and you think to yourself, "He's spineless!" When we label other people like this, we're taking just a fragment of their behavior and turning it into a personality defect. No one's behavior is *always* bad (or *always* good, for that matter), so labels are illogical. What's more, labels lead us to become angry and frustrated with the person. Everything he or she does starts to seem colored by the label, and we become more and more judgmental, causing interpersonal problems and more stress.

Graham's mother-in-law, a schoolteacher, liked to talk about her students . . . *incessantly*. She had a way of leading most conversations back to this topic, which occasionally got on Graham's nerves. But it was when he stuck her with a negative label—"She's an annoying *person*"—that the real trouble started. Graham began to notice more and more little things his mother-in-law said and did that got under his skin. He ignored all her nice gestures and even lost sight of the fact that her behavior was harmless. It got to the point that even being in the same room as his mother-in-law triggered a stress response: increased muscle tension, heart rate, and irritability, and a strong urge to leave. Finally, Graham began criticizing his mother-in-law out loud, which caused tension between him and his wife and made his stress worse.

Now let's see if you can identify the type of stress-related thinking pattern (or patterns) associated with the following thoughts. Write the correct pattern in the blank after each example in the worksheet on the next page.

So, your beliefs, thoughts, and assumptions have a lot to do with how stressed you become in different situations. And while many potentially stressful events are beyond our control—a snowstorm, for example—you *can* control your perceptions of and reactions to these stressors (or at least you can *learn* to do so) to control your stress response. But just because you *can* control your thinking doesn't mean it's your fault that you have the kinds of thoughts that create stress. Your belief system is part of a long-standing pattern that's not easy to change. So, don't blame yourself—it only adds to the stress. Instead, understand that with practice you'll learn how to change these kinds of thoughts, attitudes, and beliefs and reduce your stress levels. You'll learn and practice these important skills when you get to Chapter 8.

IDENTIFYING STRESS-RELATED THINKING PATTERNS

1. Ed had been with the company for a long time, but his new boss wasn't giving him the same latitude that his old boss had. "He should give me more respect," Ed thought.

   Thinking pattern: _____

2. Carol has HIV. She's convinced that she'll die within a year and decides to withdraw from social activities. "What's the point of HIV support groups?" she tells herself. "It's hopeless. My life is over. I can't enjoy anything anymore."

   Thinking pattern: _____

3. Valentine's Day is coming up, and Sara is alone. She's frustrated. "I can't stand it! Everyone else is happy because they have someone to be with, but I have no one."

   Thinking pattern: _____

4. Rick's travel agency is having trouble staying afloat these days. He's worried about providing for his family. "I'm a failure as a husband and father," he tells himself.

   Thinking pattern: _____

5. Amanda was an excellent lawyer, but she was constantly worried. "What if a client finds a mistake that I made and decides to sue me? What if I lose my license and get disbarred!?"

   Thinking pattern: _____

Next, try to think of some personal examples of your own stress-related thinking patterns. Choose five situations from the lists of stressful life events and daily hassles you read through earlier in this chapter. Describe the situation (A) and your thinking pattern (B) below.

1. Situation (A): _____

   Thoughts (B's): _____

2. Situation (A): _____

   Thoughts (B's): _____

3. Situation (A): _____

   Thoughts (B's): _____

4. Situation (A): _____

   Thoughts (B's): _____

5. Situation (A): _____

   Thoughts (B's): _____

IDENTIFYING YOUR C's: NEGATIVE EMOTIONS

Strong negative emotions that result from stressful situations and thinking patterns exacerbate stress because they get you off your game plan for dealing with your stressors. Anxiety, depression, and anger are emotional states that sap your ability to concentrate and see the world logically. In addition, these feelings are usually accompanied by disruptive behaviors that interfere with coping and just make matters worse. In this section, you'll identify your own levels of anxiety, depression, and anger and determine whether it's worth getting extra help for these problems beyond what is offered in this workbook.

Anxiety

Stress and anxiety are closely related—most people who have one also have the other. Anxiety is the emotion that occurs when you perceive that you're in danger but feel that you can't do anything about it. The danger could be anything from physical harm to committing a social blunder and feeling embarrassed. And the threat doesn't have to be real—anxiety results from the *perception* of danger. You might jump to conclusions about an upcoming event, such as meeting an important work or school deadline, and be unable to get it out of your mind. Preoccupied, you begin worrying (awfulizing), and negative thoughts race through your mind. You feel your heart start to race, your muscles tense, and you become irritable. You snap at people, lose concentration, and soon you're feeling like you've lost control.

Anxiety is exaggerated fear and worry that is unproductive, painful, and gets in the way of your life.

Concern is appropriate unease or apprehension that helps you cope better with unpleasant situations.

There's a difference between anxiety—as described above—and being *concerned*. Concern means having a moderate, appropriate degree of stress, which keeps you alert and helps you rise to the occasion and solve problems. Full-blown anxiety, on the other hand, is unproductive. It leads only to thinking and acting desperately without bothering to check out whether your catastrophic perceptions are really accurate.

What's your level of anxiety? Using the scale from 0 to 3 below, circle the number that corresponds to how often you've been bothered by each of the following anxiety-related problems over the past two weeks.

0 = Not at all   1 = Several days   2 = More than half the days   3 = Nearly every day

1. Feeling nervous, anxious, or on edge	0	1	2	3
2. Being unable to stop or control worrying	0	1	2	3

3. Worrying too much about different things	0	1	2	3
4. Having trouble relaxing	0	1	2	3
5. Being so restless that it is hard to sit still	0	1	2	3
6. Becoming easily annoyed or irritable	0	1	2	3
7. Feeling afraid, as if something awful might happen	0	1	2	3

Simply add up your answers to determine your score on this scale. What's your total? If it's 7 or greater, you're experiencing at least a moderate degree of anxiety. Is your score 15 or more? If so, your stress levels might rise to the point of an anxiety *disorder* such as generalized anxiety disorder, social phobia, or panic disorder (defined more specifically in Chapter 2). In addition to working through this book, I recommend seeking out a qualified clinical psychologist who can evaluate you to see if professional help would be beneficial. Most anxiety problems can be managed with cognitive-behavioral therapy (CBT). You can read about anxiety disorders and the proper form of treatment at *www.adaa.org* (the website of the Anxiety and Depression Association of America).

Depression

Some people who are stressed or anxious and feeling that the world is a dangerous place that can't be controlled lose hope and slip into a state of depression. People who experience depression feel down in the dumps more often than not because they view themselves as worthless (labeling) and the future as bleak (jumping to conclusions). They also lose interest in activities and people they once enjoyed.

Depression is different from sadness or disappointment, which are a normal part of life. When you're sad or disappointed, you're able to get back on track after a little while, think things through, and realize that the unpleasant situation will pass with time. When you're depressed, however, you don't feel motivated to help yourself. You can't focus on anything but the negative side of yourself and the future. You blame yourself for everything and feel as if you're carrying the weight of the world on your shoulders. You might also have crying spells, lose your appetite, have trouble sleeping, become socially isolated, and perhaps have thoughts of harming yourself.

Do you have problems with depression? Using the scale from 0 to 3, circle the number that corresponds to how often you've been bothered by each of the following problems over the past two weeks.

0 = Not at all   1 = Only occasionally   2 = Often   3 = Almost always

1. I feel hopeless, like I can't do anything right.	0	1	2	3
2. I feel helpless, like the future is bleak.	0	1	2	3

3. I blame myself when things go wrong.	0	1	2	3
4. I feel so unhappy that I feel like crying.	0	1	2	3
5. I have thoughts of harming or killing myself.	0	1	2	3
6. I can laugh and see the funny side of things.	0	1	2	3
7. I look forward to things I usually enjoy.	0	1	2	3

The first step in scoring this scale is to reverse your answers to questions 6 and 7. So, if you circled 0 on either of these items, your score is actually 3. If you circled 1, give yourself a score of 2. A score of 2 becomes 1. And if you answered 3 on either of these items, your score becomes 0. Once you've reversed your scores for questions 6 and 7 (only), you're ready to add up your responses. What's your total score? If it's 7 or greater, you're likely experiencing at least some feelings of depression, guilt, loss, and extreme sadness. Was your total score 15 or higher? If so, you might be experiencing clinical levels of depression that require professional help. It might be worth getting in touch with a psychologist or psychiatrist who can evaluate you for a mood disorder and discuss treatment options. There are effective treatments for depression. You can read about these at *www.abct.org* (the website for the Association for Behavioral and Cognitive Therapies).

Anger

Anger is another basic human emotion that we all experience from time to time. It occurs when we perceive that we have been purposely mistreated, disrespected, injured, or challenged or when we are faced with obstacles that keep us from meeting our personal goals. When we become angry, feelings of hostility boil to the surface and we have urges to act aggressively and destructively. Anger can lead to violence and alienate you from friends, coworkers, and family members, who might come to see you as dangerous or a "loose cannon." But people differ in how easily they become angry, the intensity of their anger, what they do when they're angry, and how long their angry spells last. Having very strict personal "rules" or "standards" for how others *must* behave and how situations *should* play out is often associated with anger problems, especially if you feel you *can't stand it* when these rules aren't followed. After all, in the real world we can't always expect people to do what we want when we want it.

While out-of-control anger leads to emotions and behaviors that intensify stress, mild

Having rigid rules for how you and others must or should behave is a recipe for stress. When these rules are inevitably broken (by you or another person—accidentally or intentionally), you end up feeling angry.

anger, such as temporarily feeling peeved or annoyed, can help you deal with stress. That's because short-term mild anger helps you stay focused and assertive—rather than aggressive—with other people. In Chapter 6 you'll learn how to manage stress using assertiveness skills.

Do you have problems with anger? Using the scale from 0 to 3, circle the number that corresponds to how often you've had each of these following problems over the past month.

0 = Not at all   1 = Rarely   2 = Occasionally   3 = Fairly often (every day or every few days)

1. I got angry and flew off the handle.	0	1	2	3
2. I had heated arguments with people close to me.	0	1	2	3
3. I was so tense with anger and frustration that I felt like I was going to explode.	0	1	2	3
4. I got angry and blurted out things that I later regretted saying.	0	1	2	3
5. I became physically violent (toward other people or things) because of my temper.	0	1	2	3
6. I had trouble forgiving people who did things I didn't like.	0	1	2	3
7. I felt as if I needed to get even with someone.	0	1	2	3

To calculate your score on this scale, all you need to do is add up your answers. What's your total? If it's 7 or greater, your stress-related thinking patterns are leading to anger. Is your score 15 or more? If so, learning to manage your anger with the help of a professional might be a good idea.

MOVING ON TO CHAPTER 4

Now that you have identified the various situational, thinking, and emotional sources of stress, you're ready to develop your game plan for reducing your stress. In Chapter 4 you'll learn about what it will take to be successful and explore the various techniques and skills available to you. You'll customize a stress management plan by matching up the sources of your stress with the treatment techniques covered in Part II. You'll also troubleshoot potential roadblocks that most people deal with when thinking about getting started on managing stress. So, turn the page . . . let's get rolling!

4

What Can You Do
about the Stress in Your Life?

Ilene was at her wit's end. An elementary school teacher, she had trouble leaving her work at work. Ilene often stayed up late at night planning the "perfect" lesson and making sure she graded her papers perfectly. She blamed herself when her students had academic or behavioral troubles. Lately she'd been losing sleep over an argument she'd had with another teacher. And when Ilene tried to smooth things over, she impulsively said some insulting things that made the situation even worse. As if her work stress wasn't enough, Ilene's family situation was also stressful. She and her husband were spending less time together these days. Were they still in love? And Ilene's daughter, Annie, was moving to Australia with her boyfriend. Ilene had always been very close with Annie, and she knew it wouldn't be easy having her so far away. All of this stress was affecting Ilene in different ways. Aside from her sleeping difficulties, she had developed a cough that never seemed to go away fully. She also tended to get nasty when she was anxious and stressed, sometimes impulsively shouting at people and calling them names. She felt lethargic and sapped of energy and was having mood swings.

Ilene had considered talking with a therapist about her stress before. She even had a pile of referral information and self-help books. Every time she got something new to read, she would vow to try to make some real changes in her life, and she'd start out determined to stick with it. But she always quickly started ruminating about how much time, energy, and money it would take to get rid of her stress. Could she really do it? After all, one of the reasons she was under so much stress was that she already had so much on her plate—worries, responsibilities, and hassles. Would this just add to them? On one hand she understood the benefits of doing something about stress. But on the other, she'd never seemed to be able to muster the energy to deal with it before. And after all, she was getting by. Her class had even won a prize for perfect attendance earlier that school year.

HAVING MIXED FEELINGS IS NORMAL

If you're like most people, then like Ilene, you probably have misgivings about managing your stress, especially if you've tested the waters before and always backed off. Sure, it would be nice to reduce your stress level. But what will you have to give up? Will reducing your stress mean settling for something less than perfection in reaching your goals? Many people feel like they need high stress in their life—like they thrive on it. And even if you don't feel that way, if you feel overwhelmed, will stress management efforts be just one more obligation?

These kinds of mixed feelings about working on stress are normal. We call them *ambivalence*—the state of having opposing positive and negative feelings *at the same time.* You view your stress as a problem, but at the same time feel you might not achieve as much without it. You're fed up with how stress is ruining your life, yet also believe that it's beyond your control. You realize you've got to do something about stress, but where will you find the time? It's like you're "on the fence."

Deciding to make changes is really tough when you're ambivalent, because you have no way of ensuring that the trade-offs will be acceptable to you. This is why it's so important to examine the pros and cons of change before you begin. When you examine your ambivalence, you'll have a better idea of what's holding you back or might stand in your way of success. You can challenge preconceived notions about what the trade-offs might mean, and you can make plans to clear away obstacles that have thwarted any efforts to change that you've made in the past.

HOW DO YOU CURRENTLY MANAGE STRESS?

The fact that you're reading this book means that whatever strategies you're currently using to manage stress are probably not working too well. Here's a checklist of different strategies people use when things get stressful. Put a check mark next to the ones that you find yourself using often.

Common Stress Management Strategies

- ❒ 1. I go to a store or online and buy things that make me feel better.
- ❒ 2. I do something such as working on a hobby or interest of mine.
- ❒ 3. I smoke or drink (alcohol or caffeine).
- ❒ 4. I exercise.
- ❒ 5. I ignore the problem and hope it goes away.
- ❒ 6. I try to put the problem in perspective.
- ❒ 7. I avoid people and just want to be alone with my problems.
- ❒ 8. I meditate, become spiritual, or try to relax myself in other ways.
- ❒ 9. I make myself feel better by eating foods that taste good.
- ❒ 10. I take a time-out and try to regroup before going back to the situation.

☐ 11. I sleep more than I need to.

☐ 12. I use humor to temporarily take the edge off.

☐ 13. I try to get other people to change their behavior that I don't like.

☐ 14. I try to focus on things I can control and just accept those that I can't.

☐ 15. I just put my head down and work as hard as I can, even if it makes me feel more stressed.

☐ 16. I confront the source of stress and see if there's anything I can do about it.

☐ 17. I take pills to calm me down or to sleep better.

Give yourself a pat on the back for all the even-numbered strategies you marked. These tend to be healthy and productive ways of dealing with stress. How many odd-numbered strategies did you mark off? Unfortunately, these tend to be less productive—sometimes seeming to work in the short term but then leading to more stress down the line. If you tend to use the odd-numbered tactics more often than not, you'll want to read the rest of this chapter carefully. Next we'll look at the pros and cons of stress, as well as the pros and cons of learning more constructive methods of managing it.

THE PROS AND CONS OF STRESS

Let's be honest: even though you realize that stress is potentially dangerous—even life threatening in high doses—you probably see some benefits to your stress. Maybe it feels like high levels of stress keep you motivated to achieve at a high level at work or school. Do you worry that your work would suffer without enough stress? Do you feel it's useful for you to assume the worst (awfulizing) in situations so that you'll always be prepared for the worst case? Are you so used to stress that you don't know what you'd do without it?

Your efforts to make changes will succeed only when you realize that your reasons for changing outweigh your reasons for not changing. It's that simple.

Ilene held some of these beliefs, and when she considered all of the advantages (pros) and disadvantages (cons) of stress, she came up with the lists in the table on the next page. As you read her pros and cons, try to think of what you'd put in your own lists.

So, what are the advantages and disadvantages of stress for *you*? Fill in the worksheet below Ilene's with your own lists.

Now review your lists. Which is longer? If there are more disadvantages than advantages of stress, you probably feel pretty committed to making some changes. On the other hand, if the lists are about even, or if the advantages of stress outweigh the disadvantages, it might be hard for you to stay motivated and be successful with this workbook. The next exercises are especially for you.

ADVANTAGES AND DISADVANTAGES OF STRESS: ILENE

Advantages of stress for me	Disadvantages of stress for me
1. It pushes me to get all my work done on time.	1. It interferes with my friendships.
2. It makes me a better teacher.	2. I get sick a lot.
3. It's comforting that I have good self-discipline.	3. It leads to arguments with my husband.
	4. I lose too much sleep.
	5. I have a hard time relaxing, even if I want to.

ADVANTAGES AND DISADVANTAGES OF STRESS

Advantages of stress for me	Disadvantages of stress for me

WHAT DOES STRESS COST YOU?

If your list of advantages is longer than your list of disadvantages, it might appear that stress isn't that big a deal for you. Yet you've bothered to read this far in a book on managing stress. Something must be wrong with this picture. So, let's take a step back and thoroughly consider the pros and cons. Here is a list of emotional, physical, social, financial, and practical consequences of being overly stressed. Think about each one and put a mark in the box next to those that apply to you.

Emotional Consequences

❐ Anxiety, panic, or extreme worry

❐ Depression, guilt, crying, or feelings of worthlessness

❐ Dissatisfaction with life

❐ Insecurity

❐ Feeling lonely or like no one understands you

❐ Outbursts of anger or constantly feeling irritable

❐ Other emotional consequences: _____

Physical Consequences

❐ Trouble sleeping or problems staying awake during the day

❐ Heart palpitations

❐ Frequent headaches, backaches, cramps, or other types of chronic pain

❐ Stomach distress (frequent indigestion, nausea, constipation, diarrhea)

❐ Weight fluctuations (extreme gains or losses)

Social Consequences

❐ Arguments and other problems with family relationships

❐ Problems at work or school

❐ Trouble enjoying social or leisure activities

❐ Using alcohol, drugs, or smoking to cope

❐ Other social consequences: _____

Financial Consequences

❐ Missed days of work

❐ Unemployment or underemployment

❐ Money spent on doctor visits or medications for stress-related problems such as anxiety, depression, or medical problems

❐ Money spent on alcohol, drugs, cigarettes, and other ways of coping with stress

❐ Other financial costs: _____

Practical Consequences

❑ Difficulty sleeping

❑ Problems with sexual functioning

❑ Problems with traveling (specify: _____)

❑ Chronic lateness

❑ Avoidance of activities you would like to do (going to parties, eating out)

❑ Avoidance of certain people or places

❑ Avoidance of routine activities such as driving, shaking hands, opening doors, reading certain books, and watching certain TV programs or movies

❑ Other practical consequences: _____

Now, with these consequences in mind, answer the questions in the worksheet on the facing page to help you identify disadvantages of being overly stressed and think about reasons for making some changes. Again, this activity will be most beneficial if you actually write down your answers rather than just thinking about them.

Now that you've thought more carefully about the negative consequences of stress, it's time to reconsider the advantages and disadvantages. Hopefully, you've realized you picked up this book for a reason: your high stress is actually more of a burden than a benefit. Wouldn't it be great if your life wasn't burdened by these negative consequences?

WHAT ARE YOUR FEELINGS ABOUT WORKING ON STRESS?

Because of her inability to commit to trying stress management in the past, Ilene was "on the fence" about doing anything about her stress. Naturally, she had some good reasons for learning stress management skills; but then she also had reasons for not wanting to do anything that felt like it might just mean more work for her. Ilene listed her reasons for and against starting a stress management program so she could see them on paper and consider them carefully. Her lists appear on page 69. Take a look at them before reading on.

Ilene's lists show that she had a number of reasons for *and* against working on stress; though she had more reasons for working on it than for choosing not to do so. What about you? Use the worksheet titled "My Feelings about Working on Stress" on page 69 to find out. On the left side of the worksheet, write down your reasons for working on stress. Then, on the right side, list your reasons for *not* doing so. If you need help coming up with ideas, take another look at Ilene's lists.

So, which list is longer? If you have more reasons *for* working on stress, keeping those in mind can help keep you on track throughout this workbook. If you have more reasons for *not* getting to work, maybe the exercise in the next section will help.

DISADVANTAGES OF TOO MUCH STRESS

Begin by writing down five things that bother you most about your problems with stress. These might be items from the checklists you just reviewed, or they might be new things you think of.

1. _____

2. _____

3. _____

4. _____

5. _____

Next, think about how these five things interfere with different areas of your life. First, how have they disrupted your social life?

- How do they get in the way of friendships, dating, or intimacy?

- How do they get in the way of activities with other people?

Describe in your own words how stress impacts your social and romantic relationships:

_____

_____

_____

Next, think about how they've interfered with your physical health.

- Do you get lots of headaches or other pains?

- Do you get sick a lot or visit the doctor often?

- What are your sleeping habits like? Are you tired a lot during the day?

- Do you eat in response to stress? Have you gained weight or had problems losing weight?

_____

_____

_____

(cont.)

DISADVANTAGES OF TOO MUCH STRESS (cont.)

Third, how have the five most bothersome aspects of stress impacted your family life?

- Do you feel tense or hostile or have many arguments with relatives?

- How do these problems keep you from reaching your full potential as a spouse or partner, parent, grandparent, son, daughter, sibling?

- How do they interfere with family activities such as celebrating holidays or vacations?

- How do your family members feel about these problems?

_____

_____

_____

Fourth, how do these five aspects of stress affect your performance at work or school?

- Do you have trouble with deadlines?

- Have you lost a job or had to switch jobs because of stress?

- Have you had to miss work or school because of stress-related problems?

- How have these issues stifled your performance at work or your grades in school?

_____

_____

_____

Last, but not least, how does stress affect you financially?

- Has it led to unemployment or being passed over for promotions?

- Do you buy things when you're stressed to make you feel better, or spend money on things such as alcohol, drugs, or tobacco products?

- How else has stress been a financial burden?

_____

_____

_____

MY FEELINGS ABOUT WORKING ON STRESS: ILENE

Reasons to work on stress	Reasons *not* to work on stress
• *I want my relationship with my husband to be better.* • *I want to have control over my life.* • *I want to be able to sleep better.* • *I could be myself again.* • *I spend too much time worried about things that are probably not that big a deal.* • *My work relationships would be a lot richer if I didn't have problems with stress.* • *Stress makes me feel bad about myself and makes me feel panicky and anxious.* • *My stress gets in the way of too many things and keeps me from enjoying myself.*	• *It's too hard. I won't be successful. I've been like this for too long.* • *Stress keeps me from making mistakes.* • *I can get by with the way things are now.* • *I don't have the time to devote to it.* • *I don't want to give in to everyone who tells me I need help.*

MY FEELINGS ABOUT WORKING ON STRESS

Reasons to work on stress	Reasons *not* to work on stress

WHAT WILL YOU GET OUT OF STRESS MANAGEMENT?

To be successful at managing stress you'll have to invest lots of time, effort, and hard work. What can you expect in return for your investment? For one thing, reducing stress can improve your physical health—in both the short and long term. The techniques in this workbook can also improve your relationships with others as well as your work or school performance and personal accomplishments. Last but not least, you'll develop more self-confidence and self-esteem and be more satisfied with life.

So, how would your life be different if you weren't constantly battling anxiety, depression, guilt, anger, or medical issues associated with stress? What would you do if you felt more confident about dealing with difficult situations in your life? What would you accomplish if you slept better at night and calmed your body and mind? Think about these questions and write on the following blanks several ways your life would be better without so much stress in the picture:

_____

_____

_____

Next, think about your physical health. Have you visited the doctor recently? Is your health a concern? Do you have chronic medical problems? Do you have a significant risk for a particular type of illness or a family history of a particular type of illness? How would it feel if you knew you were reducing the risk of illness by taking stress out of the equation? Describe how reducing your stress could improve your health on the blanks that follow:

_____

_____

_____

How do your issues with stress affect the significant others in your life? Do these people act negatively toward you? Do you have lots of arguments? Describe on the following lines how your relationships with important people in your life would improve if you weren't so stressed:

_____

_____

_____

At this point you've explored disadvantages of the status quo and advantages of making changes. Perhaps you've found that you had concrete, valid reasons for picking up this book—that you could be better off in lots of ways if you worked on learning strategies for managing stress. But stress management, like stress itself, is multifaceted. The recipe for success is to have lots of tricks up your sleeve. You'll also need to know how to use these strategies appropriately. The rest of this chapter will help you think about your goals for stress management and identify the techniques best suited to reaching these goals.

GOALS OF STRESS MANAGEMENT

Remember from Chapter 1 that stress is not all bad. In fact, you need a certain amount to do your best—whether it's in school, at work, on the ball field, when making important decisions, or in your interactions with other people. So, it shouldn't surprise you that the goal of managing stress is *not* to eliminate all stress. Life would get pretty boring without some changes or challenges from time to time. And remember that some sources of stress are *positive* events that we wouldn't want to do away with: weddings, promotions, births, building that new dream house, and so on. Most important, though, it would be impossible to eliminate all sources of stress—and *stress* itself for that matter.

So, what *is* the goal? That depends on things such as the nature of your individual stressors, your personal situation, personality style, and priorities. In general, though, the goal of stress management is to help you learn to regulate your stress level so that *you* can choose how much you need based on your circumstances, personality, and priorities. Ultimately, this will help you maximize your performance and your personal satisfaction. You can achieve this goal by using a blend of helpful strategies for problem solving, communicating more effectively, managing your time more efficiently, reducing the influences of stress-inducing maladaptive thoughts and beliefs (B's), and learning to relax your body and mind. By learning about and practicing using these tools, you'll learn how to cope effectively with the stressors in your life.

What You Can and Can't Change

As I've mentioned, some situations that provoke stress can be controlled by directly confronting and changing one of their aspects so that the situation becomes less stressful. For example, let's say you're extremely stressed because you have several work or school projects due at the same time. To change the situation you could ask your boss or teacher for an extension, which would solve the problem and reduce some of your stress.

But there are other sources of stress that you just can't change, such as a serious illness or a death in the family. It can also be very difficult to get people to change their behavior. And even in the deadline extension example you just read, simply because you *ask* for an extension doesn't mean it will be granted. So, the reality is that while we can *try* to change some stressful situations, this won't work all the time. That's why it's very important to have a back-up plan just in case there's not much you can do about the situation itself. It turns out that the best back-up plan is learning how to correct exaggerated or maladaptive thoughts and beliefs (B's) about these difficult situations that make them seem worse than they really are. Remember Jamie and Melissa from Chapter 2? When there was nothing they could do about the snowstorm that grounded their plane, Melissa was able to control her stress because of how she thought about the situation. Jamie, on the other hand, became extremely stressed because she believed it was a true catastrophe.

*Although you **can't** always change the situation, you **can** change how you think about it.*

Let's consider some different types of stressors and how best to approach managing them. For each type, think about the degree to which you might be better off working to change the situation itself, versus changing the way you *think about* the situation.

Work- and School-Related Stressors

Do you spend more time at work (or school) than at home? Many people do. And for most of us, these are very important parts of our lives. So, it's not surprising that they can be major sources of stress. It turns out that you might be able to change (or at least try to change) some work or school stressors. If, for example, you have flexible supervisors or teachers, it might be possible to get extra help, a break on a work project, or deadline extensions for turning work in. But if your supervisor or teacher is less flexible, you might not catch such breaks even if you ask. If you're having problems with budgeting your time, you can learn time management skills. If studying for exams stresses you out, you could attend a study skills session or find a tutor.

Are you stressed about disagreements, office politics, peer pressure, or other interpersonal issues with supervisors, coworkers, peers, or teachers? Learning effective communication strategies can sometimes help you get the other person to see things your way—but not always. So, it's never a helpful strategy to expect that unpleasant coworker, peer, or professor to change his or her behavior just to suit you. If you aren't successful with changing the stressful situation directly, you'll need to reduce your stress by changing how you think about the situation (like Melissa in Chapter 3).

Interpersonal Stressors

Dealing with people—family members, coworkers, authority figures, friends—is an important part of almost every day. So it's no wonder that not getting along well with others can lead to a great deal of stress. Dealing with interpersonal stressors involves discovering your own set of coping mechanisms. As I already mentioned, on the one hand you might be able to change or avoid some of these stressors. For instance, you can break up with a verbally abusive boyfriend or simply avoid that clingy "friend" who won't leave you alone when you're trying to study. You can explain to your confrontational father-in-law that you prefer not to discuss religion and politics with him anymore and get couple therapy if you're having frequent disagreements with your spouse or partner. However, because you can't expect other people to change for you, you'll also need to be able to reduce your stress by changing your expectations of others and thinking in ways that keep your negative emotions in check.

Financial Stressors

Financial strain also happens to be among the most common sources of stress. There might be little you can do about stock market losses or a failed business venture. And being in debt or unable to afford things that you want can be extremely stressful, though there's not always much you can do about it right away. There might be things you can do to gradually change your financial situation, such as changing your spending habits and working with a financial adviser; but this may take time, and learning to think about your financial situation in a healthy way will be important. If you and your spouse or partner argue about how to spend your money, which often leads to stress, this too can often be dealt with through problem solving, effective communication, and perhaps assistance from a therapist or financial adviser.

Daily Hassles

Traffic, a broken home appliance, a sick child, bad weather—there is little we can do to change or avoid many of these problems. They often happen when we least expect it, catching us off guard. But sometimes we blow them out of proportion. So, you'll need to learn how not to make mountains out of these molehills. Still, there are hassles that you *can* sometimes avoid or change. Don't like to sit in traffic? Choose a different route or time to travel. Do your kids get the flu every winter? Perhaps the flu shot or other preventive health measures would help. Problem-solving strategies along with helpful thinking skills are often a good one–two punch for managing stress that comes from daily hassles.

Major Life Events

Stressors in this category include events that change your life in significant ways. They're often unpleasant or unfortunate events such as the death of a loved one, a serious accident or injury, illness, loss of a job, divorce, living with the constant threat of crime, and the like. As much as we'd like to prevent such situations, they might be unavoidable. Certain positive life-changing events also fall within this category: having a baby, getting married, and taking a new job. Once they occur, it's very difficult (or impossible) to change their course. So, whether it's a crisis or a cause for celebration, it's how we think about an event that determines how much stress we experience. In Chapter 8, you'll learn how

EYE ◗PENER

A Fail-Safe Approach to Stress Management

Although it might be worth trying to intervene in, avoid, or change some stress-provoking situations, this is not always possible. Yet, as you read in Chapter 3, extreme stress is associated with exaggerated, maladaptive thoughts and belief systems. So, even when you can't make the stressful situation go away, you can reduce your stress by changing your thinking so it's less exaggerated and more adaptive. The beauty of mastering this approach is that it means that *you* will always have the ultimate control over stress and your emotions. No matter what happens to you—negative events, unpleasant situations, disrespectful people, and the like—if all else fails, you'll still be able to regulate your stress level by controlling how you think.

to identify maladaptive thinking patterns and change them so that they don't lead to so much stress.

Matching Your Stressors with Stress-Reduction Methods

Now it's time to figure out which of the techniques in this workbook are best suited for managing the sources of stress in your life. Because everyone responds differently to stressors, I can't say for sure which techniques will work best for you, but this section is designed to get you started with a solid stress-reduction plan. The first step is to become familiar with the six stress management strategies that are covered in Part II of this workbook (I've already hinted at some of them throughout this chapter). They're briefly described in the chart on the facing page.

Now that you have an idea of the techniques we'll use to defuse stress, the next step is to identify the top five sources of stress in your life. You might take a look back at the checklists of stress producers from Chapter 3. Once you know what they are, write them down on the lines that follow.

My Top Sources of Stress:

1. _____

2. _____

3. _____

4. _____

5. _____

Next, take a look at the chart on page 76. It gives you an idea of the most effective stress-reduction techniques for different types of stressors and includes spaces for you to

Stress Management Techniques

Technique	Chapter	Description
Problem solving	5	Learning how to identify problems, generate solutions, make decisions, and implement plans to cope with stressful situations
Communication/assertiveness skills	6	Learning to improve assertiveness and negotiation skills to gain confidence in yourself and respect from others
Time management	7	Learning skills for boosting your personal efficiency and productivity
Cognitive restructuring	8	Learning to identify and correct exaggerated, distorted, and maladaptive thinking patterns that lead to stress responses
Muscle relaxation and meditation	9	Learning and practicing skills for activating the relaxation response even in the midst of a stressful situation and for calming yourself by freeing your mind from stress and worrisome thoughts
Maintaining a healthy lifestyle	10	Maximizing good health habits such as eating healthily, getting exercise, and sleeping well

write in your own stressors that you identified on the previous page. The techniques are listed across the top of the chart, and sources of stress are listed down the left side. Don't worry if your stressful events don't fit neatly into one of the categories in the chart—that's why I included space for writing in your own. Also, notice that more than one technique can be helpful for each type of stressor. I've marked one or more technique(s) that are likely to be most effective for a given stressor with a ▲. Other helpful techniques for dealing with that particular type of stressor are indicated by a △. Of course, you'll get the best results by applying all of the indicated strategies.

As you can see, cognitive restructuring is helpful for all types of stressors. That's because this is the technique that will help you correct the exaggerated, maladaptive thoughts and belief systems (the B's from Chapter 3) that lead to stress and negative emotions. Remember, it's the one technique that helps alleviate stress even when you can't change or avoid the stressful situation. For that reason, I strongly recommend spending time working on learning cognitive restructuring skills in Chapter 8.

Notice also that maintaining a healthy lifestyle is recommended for all types of stressors. And while being healthy is not, by itself, going to get rid of your stressors, it will give you an edge on dealing with stress in both the short term and the long run. In the short term, when you eat right, get exercise, and sleep well, you'll feel better and have

RECOMMENDED STRESS MANAGEMENT TECHNIQUE(S)

Source of stress	Problem solving (Chapter 5)	Communication/ assertiveness skills (Chapter 6)	Time management (Chapter 7)	Cognitive restructuring (Chapter 8)	Muscle relaxation (Chapter 9)	Meditation (Chapter 9)	Maintaining a healthy lifestyle (Chapter 10)
Major life event				▲	△	△	△
Daily hassles	△			▲	△	△	△
Interpersonal stressors	△	▲		▲		△	△
Financial stressors	▲			▲		△	△
Work (and school) stressors	△	△	▲	△			△
Work–life balance issues	▲	△	△	△	△	△	△
1.							
2.							
3.							
4.							
5.							

more physical and mental energy for dealing successfully with stressors. And given what you now know about the long-term effects of stress on your health, it should be clear that investing the time and energy now to optimize and maintain a healthy lifestyle will pay off big-time later in life.

Now, before moving on, complete the chart on the facing page by writing in your top five sources of stress in the numbered rows. Which stress management techniques will you focus on to deal with these stressors? Moving across each row, place a mark in the box for each technique that you feel would be helpful. This chart can serve as your road map as you embark on your stress-management journey.

Armed and Ready

Now that you're an expert on stress, how it affects you, and what you can do about it—and now that you have a game plan—you're ready to take action. Move on to Part II and begin trying out the various strategies you identified as looking helpful. In Part III, I'll help you use these techniques with some particularly common types of stressors. Just keep the following in mind as you work through Part II: like any skill, learning to use stress management techniques requires patience and practice. Take your time—it's worth investing your time and energy right now in order to have a less stressful future.

Part II

Reducing Your Stress

5

Solving the Problems in Your Life

Problems ranging from daily hassles (your child is sick and can't go to school, but *you* can't stay home from work) to major life crises (your spouse loses his job) are a part of life. Yet even greater stress results when ongoing problems (your teenager's glued to the computer screen 24/7) remain unsolved or are solved in unproductive ways (yell, harass, but never approach him with consistent resolve). As you've learned, feeling like you don't have control over a challenging situation causes significant stress. One approach is what psychologists term "structured problem solving." This approach gives you back a sense of control and may even eliminate some problems entirely. In this chapter, you'll learn the steps for identifying problems, generating possible solutions, and carrying out action plans.

The strategies are derived from structured problem-solving therapy, an approach that is well researched and used extensively in stress management programs. Will you be able to use this approach to completely solve all of your problems and eliminate all stressful situations? Probably not. But when used in combination with other techniques, such as changing maladaptive thinking patterns (see Chapter 8), problem solving can help you deal with many situations that presently trigger stress.

WHAT IS PROBLEM SOLVING?

Continually obsessing about a challenging situation is a sign that you probably handle this and other problems in unproductive ways. Maybe you become fearful. Maybe you look for someone to pin the blame on. Maybe you put too much pressure on yourself to come up with the perfect solution. Maybe you try

Slow down! Solving problems is like approaching a curve in the road. Go at the right speed and you'll be in good shape for the straightaway that follows. Go too fast and you could end up in a ditch.

to ignore the problem, hoping it will just go away on its own. Regardless, when you're stressed out, being faced with a problem becomes a problem—which only compounds your stress.

The structured form of problem solving taught here will help you use your creativity to think outside the box and generate solutions you might not have thought of before. You'll analyze the problem from different angles and develop a plan for resolving it. The ultimate goal of problem solving is to find the best long-term solution. But effective problem solving can take a lot of time and effort (less time and effort than a problem that is not properly solved, though!). The key will be slowing down and working carefully. In this chapter you'll learn to problem-solve by following five steps.

The Five Steps to Effective Problem Solving

Step 1: Recognizing problems

Step 2: Choosing and clarifying a problem to solve

Step 3: Brainstorming solutions

Step 4: Narrowing down the possibilities

Step 5: Developing and carrying out an action plan

YOUR PROBLEM ORIENTATION

What are your thoughts and beliefs about problems in general? Do you think that they're somehow planted in front of you by someone else? Do you think they're irritating, but a normal part of life? Do you think they're caused by other people's behavior, but still your issue to deal with? What about your thoughts and feelings about your ability to solve them? It turns out that how you think about challenging situations, and your attitude about your ability to problem-solve, plays a large role in your response to any given problem. And that could mean the difference between successfully solving an issue at hand and letting it get the best of you. So, before we begin working on solving problems we need to determine your *problem orientation*—your feelings about problems and your capacity to solve them. To illustrate, read the stories of Harrison and Rebecca. You'll see how differently they approached having to solve problems.

Harrison's teenage son, Tyler, suffered from obsessive–compulsive disorder (OCD), but he refused to get any help. And Tyler's OCD created problems for the whole family: Everyone was required to follow certain cleaning rituals; the family was often late as a result; and Tyler often had episodes of intense anxiety and anger, which were disruptive. It seemed like the house-

hold was spinning out of control—almost everything was affected by Tyler's OCD. Harrison believed this problem needed to be confronted directly, and he was willing to take the time and effort to do so. Whether or not Tyler would agree to get help for OCD, Harrison was intent on making sure that Tyler's behavior no longer affected the family so completely. His approach illustrates a positive *problem orientation. He had the kinds of thoughts and beliefs about problems, and how to solve them, that will also help you face your problems head on and use effective skills to solve them.*

Rebecca's situation with her apartment totally stressed her out. Every few days, the bathtub from the apartment upstairs was causing floods (Rebecca later discovered that this neighbor used drugs while bathing and would routinely pass out before remembering to turn off the bath water; and the water would overflow for hours and drip through the floor and down into Rebecca's apartment!). The flooding had ruined pictures hung on Rebecca's walls, and some of her clothes, and she even had to replace her computer. As a graduate student, Rebecca didn't have a lot of money. She wanted this all to stop, but didn't know what to do. She knew she should confront her neighbor, but felt too upset to do so. Instead, she left a message with the rental office, but no one ever got back to her. Her stress rose increasingly until one morning, after yet another flood, she stormed into the rental office and screamed at the secretary. Of course, this didn't help matters. In fact, the only result was that Rebecca received a threatening letter from the landlord. Rebecca felt frustrated and drained of options. Could anything be done about this? Her set of actions illustrates a negative problem orientation—she didn't think she could resolve the issue on her own (too frightened to talk to her neighbor and hoping the landlord would intervene), which made her feel helpless and caused her to lose control and yell at the secretary in the rental office. These thoughts and beliefs kept her from using effective problem-solving strategies.

So, what's *your* problem orientation? Are you ready to start solving the problems that trigger stress in your life? The questionnaire that follows will help you figure this out. Use the following rating scale to circle the number representing how much you agree with each statement.

0 = Strongly disagree   1 = Slightly disagree   2 = Slightly agree   3 = Strongly agree

1.	I avoid problems or wait for other people to solve them for me.	0	1	2	3
2.	It's worth spending a lot of time and effort to solve a problem correctly.	0	1	2	3
3.	When problems occur, it's because there is something wrong with me.	0	1	2	3
4.	I'm capable of solving most of my problems.	0	1	2	3

5. Having to solve problems is threatening and   0   1   2   3
    upsetting.

6. I'm overwhelmed by problems that I can't solve.   0   1   2   3

7. I'm up to the challenge of solving my problems.   0   1   2   3

8. Most problems can be solved.   0   1   2   3

9. Problems are a normal part of life.   0   1   2   3

10. I'm not very good at solving problems.   0   1   2   3

The first step in scoring this questionnaire is to reverse your scores for items 1, 3, 5, 6, and 10 because these five questions are worded in the negative. So, if you had a 0 on any of these items, change that to a 3. If you had a 1, give yourself a 2. If you had a 2, give yourself a 1, and if you scored 3 on any of these items, change it to 0.

With those five items reversed, add up all 10 of your scores. Your total will be somewhere between 0 and 30. Higher scores represent a more *positive* problem orientation. In fact scoring 20 or above suggests that you understand problems are a normal part of life and you view them as challenges and opportunities to make changes for the good. Like Harrison, you're in a good place to start solving your problems. You realize it might take lots of time, effort, and persistence, but you're committed. Good for you!

If your total score is 10 or less, you might have a *negative* problem orientation. You might feel stressed out just knowing that there's a problem to be solved. You might even blame yourself for problems and doubt that you'll be able to do much about them. If you feel generally overwhelmed by your problems, then, like Rebecca, your approach to trying to solve problems is not working very well. Maybe you ignore problems, hoping they'll go away; or you rely on others to solve them for you. Perhaps you act impulsively, making snap decisions without much thought. If this sounds like you, understand that you can change your problem orientation. In fact, as you go through this chapter and learn the proper steps for healthy problem solving, it's likely that you'll develop a more positive orientation. But in the meantime, you can start by committing to memory these facts about problems and their solutions:

- "Problems are common—they're a normal part of life for everyone."

- "Solving most problems takes time and effort. I can't expect this to always be easy."

- "I can learn from dealing with problems."

- "Most problems can be solved, even if it takes time and commitment."

- "Blaming myself or others for a problem doesn't actually help to solve it."

STEP 1: RECOGNIZING PROBLEMS

It might seem obvious, but to solve a problem you need to recognize that one actually exists. Perhaps you've got a problem that's easy to spot, but it's not always so straightforward. Sometimes we just experience the negative thoughts and feelings or have physical symptoms without realizing that they are connected to a particular problem. Stress-related behaviors (such as alcohol use or general hostility) might also be a sign that an unsolved problem is festering. When you find yourself experiencing the symptoms of stress that you learned about in Chapter 1 (angry outbursts, insomnia, racing heart, self-blame, and the like), chances are there's an underlying problem that needs solving. If you know what problems you're currently experiencing, begin by describing them in the Problem List worksheet below. Then move on to step 2 of problem solving on page 88.

PROBLEM LIST

	Brief description of the problem
1.	
2.	
3.	
4.	
5.	
6.	
7.	
8.	
9.	
10.	

From *The Stress Less Workbook.* Copyright 2012 by The Guilford Press.

If you're having trouble identifying specific problems, you can use *problem cues* to help. Read on.

Identifying Problem Cues

If you feel stressed for no reason—or you're having a hard time putting your finger on a specific problem—begin by using the Problem Cues worksheet below to identify your thoughts, feelings, physical symptoms, and behaviors that could be signs of a problem.

MY PROBLEM CUES

Make a list of the various signs and symptoms you're experiencing that indicate the presence of a problem, as well as when and where they occurred.

Thoughts	Feelings	Physical symptoms	Behaviors	Day/time/ situation

From *The Stress Less Workbook*. Copyright 2012 by The Guilford Press.

MY PROBLEM CUES: REBECCA

Thoughts	Feelings	Physical symptoms	Behaviors	Day/time/ situation
• My life is a mess. • I can't do anything right. • People are out to get me.	• Angry • Powerless • Less interested in being with people	• Racing heart • Muscle tension • No appetite	• Snapping at people I care about • Wanting to be by myself more than usual • Can't sleep	• June 23 • 10:30 P.M. • Third time the apartment has flooded

Rebecca completed this worksheet (above). She'd been feeling angry a lot, which wasn't the way she usually behaved. She was even snapping at people more often, such as her mother and coworkers, who had absolutely nothing to do with her problem.

Rebecca first noticed the problem cues that she listed in her worksheet after there had been three floods in 1 week's time. She noticed that her anger got worse when the landlord's office didn't return her phone call after 3 days. You can work backwards from the problem cues to identify specific problems that triggered the cues in the same way that Rebecca did. When did you first notice your problem cues? What was happening around the time that you noticed them? After giving it some thought, Rebecca came up with the problems listed below.

- *Frequent flooding in the apartment*

- *The landlord doesn't know what's going on and isn't helping me*

- *Loss of money from paying for repairs and replacements that I didn't cause*

After you consider what problems triggered your cues, briefly describe them in the problem list on page 85 so you have some targets for using the problem-solving strategies in this chapter.

STEP 2: CHOOSING AND CLARIFYING A PROBLEM TO SOLVE

Once you have a list of one or more problems, the next step involves selecting and describing the one you want to work on. Clearly defining the problem will make it easier to find effective solutions. There's a method to choosing the right problem to start with, and clarifying it. Read on.

Guidelines for Choosing a Problem to Work On

Take a look at your problem list. Whether it's a small list or on the longer side, it's best to work on problems one at a time. But which problem should you work on first, second, third, and so on? Here are some guidelines to follow that may improve the chances of having success with your problem solving:

1. **Start with an *easy* problem.** If you start small, you'll be able to move through the problem-solving steps quickly and learn how the process works. Then you can gradually tackle larger and more challenging problems.
2. **Start with a problem that feels *manageable*.** If possible, get your feet wet with solving problems that you feel you have a greater degree of control over. Having early success with problem solving will increase your confidence in the process.
3. **Start with a *practical* problem.** It's also best to begin with a problem that's important to you and applicable in your life. In other words, a problem that will make a noticeable (although not necessarily life-changing) difference when it is solved.
4. **How *urgent* is the problem?** The easiest, most manageable, and most practical problem is not always the most pressing. But is the clock ticking? If some of your problems need solving right away, it's okay to make them a priority.

Clarifying the Target Problem

Once you've chosen a *target problem* (that is, the problem you're going to work on), it's important to examine it thoroughly and consider all the relevant facts. You also need to be objective, which means trying to understand the facts of the problem rather than focusing on your opinion or judgments about who is to blame. Spelling out the details of your problem and getting a clear sense of how it affects you will make it much easier for you to generate solutions in the next step. The Clarifying a Problem worksheet on the facing page is a tool for you to use when homing in on your target problem. Enter the target problem you're working on at the top of the worksheet and then answer each of the questions that follow. You might make blank copies of the worksheet so you can repeat this process as you take on each problem in your problem list. Take a look at Rebecca's worksheet (page 90) for an example. The problem she chose to work on first was that her landlord didn't realize she had a problem. She needed to let the landlord know before she could expect to get any help.

> *When the problem is unclear, the solution will be too.*

CLARIFYING A PROBLEM

Describe the target problem you're working on.

Why is this a problem for you (how did it become a problem, and in what ways does it affect you)?

When do you notice the problem?

How often does it occur?

Where does it occur?

Who is involved?

What have you done to try to solve this problem in the past? How do you deal with it when it comes up?

What parts of this problem *do* you have control over? What do you *not* have control over?

Other important facts about this problem:

CLARIFYING A PROBLEM: REBECCA

Describe the target problem you're working on.

The landlord and rental office don't realize that my apartment is flooding several times each week.

Why is this a problem for you (how did it become a problem, and in what ways does it affect you)?

I need help dealing with the floods because it's costing me money and stressing me out. If the landlord doesn't realize what's going on, he can't help me. It became a problem because I didn't take the proper action to let the landlord know about it sooner.

When do you notice the problem? *When I'm at home and I see the effects of the flooding.*

How often does it occur? *I'm in my apartment every morning and evening.*

Where does it occur? *My apartment*

Who is involved? *The rental office/landlord, me, my upstairs neighbor*

What have you done to try to solve this problem in the past? How do you deal with it when it comes up?

I left a voice mail message at the rental office; I went in and yelled at the secretary in the rental office. Sometimes when I'm at home and I'm thinking about this problem I get angry and think about ways to get back at the person upstairs, but I never do anything. Sometimes I just cry because I feel helpless.

What parts of this problem *do* you have control over? What do you *not* have control over?

I can control how I let the landlord know about the flooding in my apartment. I can't control what he does about it or how helpful he is. I can't control whose side he is on.

Other important facts about this problem:

The floods have ruined some of my things; I made a mistake in getting angry before; I have a lease that isn't up for another 9 months, but it's unacceptable to have frequent flooding like this.

STEP 3: BRAINSTORMING SOLUTIONS

Once you've selected and clarified your target problem, it's time to generate possible solutions. *Brainstorming* is a common enough term in business, but therapists define it specifically as a way to come up with as many possible ways of solving your problem as you can. Don't judge the solution by how effective it might be at this point; just write down as many possible solutions as you can think of. Whether it's a good or bad idea doesn't matter. It just has to be relevant to the problem and have a chance of working (or at least *helping* to solve the problem). Why should you be nonjudgmental about possible solutions at this stage? Because you want your list of ideas for solving your problem to be as long as possible. That way you increase the chances you'll come up with creative solutions.

When you brainstorm, it's helpful to be in a calm, quiet environment—or in whatever setting you do your best thinking and feel free to loosen up. Be creative, imaginative, and resourceful. Don't be afraid to come up with extreme or outrageous ideas. And you don't have to do all of your brainstorming at one time. You can always add to your list of possible solutions if an idea hits you later. You might ask other people—friends or relatives who tend to be nonjudgmental—for their ideas too. Remember, at this stage don't worry about how you're going to implement your possible solutions. Your job here is only to generate as many possibilities as you can think of. We'll narrow down your choices later.

So, as you consider your target problem, what ideas come to mind? On the next page is the Brainstorming worksheet for writing down possible ways of solving your problem. Again, make copies of this form so you can use it with each problem on your problem list. You can see the results of Rebecca's brainstorming on page 93.

STEP 4: NARROWING DOWN THE POSSIBILITIES

Now it's time to think about the advantages and disadvantages of the various solutions you came up with in your brainstorming session. Your ultimate goal in this step is to narrow the list down to possible solutions that are a good fit for dealing with your problem. It's easy to feel overwhelmed at this point, especially if you have lots of possible solutions to consider. Maybe you've pondered these options before but ended up just going round and round about them in your mind. I'll help you get beyond this mental block by giving you the guidelines and structure you'll need to choose solutions that are doable, feasible, and have a good chance of either solving the problem or helping to solve it.

Eliminating Unrealistic Solutions

Right off the bat, let's eliminate any ideas that seem unrealistic or that look like they just wouldn't work. Take a look at your Brainstorming worksheet and cross any of these off. You can also use the three guidelines at the bottom of page 93 to help you make the initial cuts:

BRAINSTORMING

Describe the target problem.

List potential solutions.

1.

2.

3.

4.

5.

6.

7.

8.

9.

10.

11.

12.

13.

14.

15.

BRAINSTORMING: REBECCA

Describe the target problem. *The landlord doesn't realize that my apartment is flooding several times each week.*

List potential solutions.

1. *Write a letter to the landlord describing what's happening*

2. *Call and schedule an appointment to meet with the landlord*

3. *Go in person to the rental office to see if the landlord is there*

4. *Find a lawyer and have him or her get in touch with the landlord for me*

5. *Ask Mom or Dad to call the rental office for me*

6. *Write a letter about the problem to the editor of the newspaper*

7. *Leave a phone message for the landlord describing what's going on*

8. *Just move to another apartment complex*

9. *E-mail the landlord and explain the problem*

10. *Call the landlord and speak with him directly*

11. *Have the landlord come to my apartment to see the damage himself*

12. *Get back at the neighbor by damaging something of his*

Guidelines for Initial Cuts to Your Brainstorming List

- **Too demanding.** Do any of your solutions require more time and money than you're realistically willing or able to spend? You can cross these off the list.

- **Too reliant on others.** Sure, your friends and relatives are willing to help you out. But the best solutions for stress-related problems are usually those where you depend mainly on yourself to do the work—that is, solutions where you're in control. No one else has your best interests in mind the way you do. And what's more, being self-reliant is an all-around important stress management skill. So, at least for now, let's eliminate solutions that rely heavily on other people acting in your stead.

- **Too harmful.** This, I hope, is an obvious one. Solutions that are likely to cause emotional or physical harm (to you or someone else) are no good. Cross them off. With solutions like these, who needs problems!?

When Rebecca reviewed her Brainstorming worksheet, she decided to cross out the idea of hiring a lawyer. After all, she was strapped for money. She also realized that this might seem overly threatening as a first step. Maybe she could save this idea for later on if other ways of getting help didn't work out. She also knew it was important to first try handling this on her own. To this end, she also eliminated the idea of asking her parents to contact the apartment complex on her behalf. Finally, she eliminated the ideas of having the landlord come to her apartment (because it involved too much reliance on someone other than herself—what if he didn't want to come?) and the idea of retaliating by causing additional property damage (two wrongs don't make a right). She did, however, add the idea of leaving her neighbor a note as a first step.

Categorizing Your Solutions

Another way to make your choice easier is to group your options together based on similar ideas. Do two or more of your potential solutions overlap? Try sorting the remaining solutions into themes so that you have *categories*, rather than individual ideas, to choose from.

When Rebecca looked over the options that remained on her brainstorming list, she was able to form three categories. Ideas #2 and #3 were very similar: both involved having a face-to-face meeting with the landlord. Ideas #1, #7, #8, and #9 were similar: they involved contacting the rental office or landlord via the phone, e-mail, or mail. Finally, option #6, writing a letter to the editor of the local newspaper, seemed to be in a category of its own.

After grouping your similar brainstorming ideas together, list your categories on the following blank lines. Rebecca's categories were (1) meet with the landlord face to face, (2) send a message to the landlord's office, and (3) write a letter to the editor.

My Solution Categories

- _____
- _____
- _____
- _____
- _____
- _____
- _____

Choosing a Possible Solution

The next step is actually choosing a category that you'd like to start with as a possible solution. Does one jump out at you as seeming like the best approach to solving your problem? Can you identify a solution by process of elimination? Choose a category and then, from within that group, choose a specific solution. Rebecca chose the group of solutions involving meeting with her landlord face to face. She also thought that scheduling a meeting ahead of time would be preferable to just showing up at the main office because she knew that the landlord often traveled to various properties he owned around town.

Evaluating Your Solution

The next part of this step is evaluating the solution you chose. It's important to determine the pros and cons—the advantages and disadvantages—of your solution before you take action. When the pros outweigh the cons, you know you've got a solution worth pursuing. If it's vice versa, you might need to go back to the drawing board. We'll also consider other key points to keep in mind that aren't necessarily advantages or disadvantages.

So, list the advantages and disadvantages of the solution you chose in the appropriate columns of the Pros and Cons of Solutions worksheet on the next page (make blank copies of this form so you can use it with additional problems and solutions). To help with this, consider the following questions when you're evaluating the solution—the pros and cons should be the answers to these questions. Any answers or ideas that are not necessarily advantages or disadvantages, but that are important to keep in mind, you can list in the "Other Key Points" column of the worksheet.

Key Questions for Evaluating Solutions

- "How feasible is this solution?"

- "How does it affect me physically and emotionally?"

- "How well does it fit with my values, goals, and other commitments in my life?"

- "How much time and effort will it require?"

- "What are the financial costs and benefits?"

- "How does it affect (physically and emotionally) the people who are close to me?"

Rebecca thought about the key questions for evaluating solutions and came up with the pros, cons, and other key points listed in her Pros and Cons of Solutions worksheet on page 97.

PROS AND CONS OF SOLUTIONS

Describe the solution: _____

Pros	Cons	Other key points

The final stage in Step 4 is to go back and actually weigh the pros and cons of the solution. The best way to do this is by reviewing your Pros and Cons worksheet and giving each pro a "+" and each con a "−." If there are pros or cons that seem especially important, you should give them two (or even three, if they're *extremely* important) pluses or minuses. Rebecca thought that feeling like she had accomplished something independently deserved two pluses, as did the fact that the meeting was so in line with her goal of letting the landlord know about the flooding. For Rebecca, the possibility of her landlord being upset was worth two minuses because she would feel very uncom-

PROS AND CONS OF SOLUTIONS: REBECCA

Describe the solution: *Schedule a meeting with the landlord to discuss the flood situation*

Pros	Cons	Other key points
• Will make me feel like I accomplished something • Requires minimal time, effort, and no financial cost • Fits my goals of needing to do something about the flooding • Doesn't hurt anyone • Seems feasible	• Landlord might be upset at me because I screamed at his secretary • Might need to adjust my schedule for this meeting • Might have to wait for an available appointment	• Need to apologize for shouting at the office staff • Need to maintain my composure in the meeting • Need to prepare what to say and how to say it

fortable if this happened. When Rebecca totaled up the pluses and minuses, her solution of scheduling an appointment to meet with the landlord had a score of +3, indicating that the pros outweighed the cons. She was ready to develop an action plan.

Rebecca's decision was relatively straightforward and easy. She had only one viable solution to consider. For some problems, though, you might have two or more possible solutions. When that's the case, you should look at the pros and cons of each option and then compare across possible solutions. If one stands out as having a much more positive score than the others, your choice is simple. If a few solutions end up having similar positive scores, then you can choose from among them. This means that you've done a great job of brainstorming. If none of the solutions you considered has a positive score (the cons outweigh the pros), you might need to choose a different category of solutions or do some more brainstorming.

STEP 5: DEVELOPING AND CARRYING OUT AN ACTION PLAN

Now it's time to put your solution(s) into action. Spending time thinking carefully about an action plan prior to acting is important for two reasons: First, it helps you break your solution down into manageable steps and create a road map to follow. Second, it can alert you to hidden obstacles that require special planning. The Action Plan worksheet on the next page walks you through the stages of developing an action plan, and the next section provides you with some tips for how to complete the worksheet and create an effective plan. Make copies of the blank worksheet so that you can reuse the form when solving other problems on your problem list.

ACTION PLAN

Describe the solution: _____

1. What needs to be done to carry out your solution?

2. What resources will you need?

3. List the steps you need to take to implement your solution and specify the date and time when you will plan to implement each step.

Step	Date/time
1.	
2.	
3.	
4.	
5.	
6.	
7.	
8.	
9.	
10.	

Use extra paper if more steps are required.

1. What needs to be done to carry out your solution? What do you need to do to put your solution into practice? Be as specific as you can. Do you need to get information about something? Do you need to ask someone for a ride somewhere? Will you need childcare? Do you need some time off from work or permission to miss class? The more detail, the better. Rebecca needed to find the phone number for the landlord's office before she could call to schedule an appointment. She also needed to look at her own schedule so she could more easily set a date and time for the meeting with her landlord. Then she needed to think about what she was going to say in the meeting. She also wanted to take some pictures of the damage in her apartment to show to her landlord.

2. What resources will you need? List the supplies that are necessary for you to execute your solution. Again, be as specific and as thorough as you can. Try to think of the little things. Do you need to get certain information from the city regarding apartment rules and regulations? Do you need a bus or train schedule? Do you need to know someone else's schedule or how much something costs? Rebecca needed to know her landlord's schedule, which she would find out when she called to set up the appointment. She also needed a digital camera for taking the pictures.

3. List the steps for implementing your solution. Breaking down larger-scale solutions into smaller, more manageable steps helps keep you from feeling overwhelmed. Following clearly planned steps toward a goal also helps keep you on track. So, write down each individual step you think you'll need to accomplish on your way to carrying out your solution. Make sure each step is *specific*—know exactly what you're going to do at each phase of the process. Make sure each is *measurable* so you can tell when you've finished each step. Each step should also be *achievable*—something you can manage given the other things that are going on in your life. Of course, all of your steps should also be *relevant* to the overall solution. There's no time for unnecessary steps when it comes to solving stressful problems!

Good action plans are also *time bound*, which means they spell out exactly when you're going to do each step—and they have a beginning and ending. This increases the chances that your problem gets solved as planned and in a timely way. It also helps you keep track of when each part of the action plan is completed. Notice that there's a column in the worksheet for you to list the specific date and time (such as Wednesday 6/11 at 5:30 P.M.) that you'll work on each part of your action plan. I suggest that you begin working on your action plan as soon as possible. The longer you wait around, the more you lose motivation or forget the reasons that you decided on this solution in the first place. Rebecca's action plan is listed below:

Rebecca's Action Plan

- *Look up the phone number to the landlord's office—Today at 3:00 after class*

- *Look at my schedule to see when I would be available to meet—Today at 3:00*

- *Call to schedule a meeting as soon as possible—Today at 3:00*

- *Prepare what I'm going to say to describe the situation—Tonight after dinner at 7:30*

- *Take pictures of the damage in my apartment to show the landlord—Tonight 8:30*

Once your action plan is in place, and you've got all the materials and resources you need to get started, begin working through the various steps. Once you've completed the action plan, you'll want to review your results to see whether the solution you used successfully resolved the problem or whether more work needs to be done. Move on to the next section after you've had a go at implementing your solution.

REVIEWING YOUR PROGRESS

Looking back and evaluating how your action plan worked is an important part of the problem-solving process because it gives you the chance to acknowledge how hard you worked and what you accomplished. It's also an opportunity to troubleshoot any unexpected bumps in the road, or other obstacles that might have gotten in the way. Sometimes when we carry out a solution, it doesn't completely solve the target problem or work exactly as we'd like. This is completely normal—especially when you're first getting started. So, if this happens to you, don't waste your time and energy taking it personally and beating up on yourself (which will only increase your stress). Instead, learn from experience and get back to work! Maybe you overlooked something when you developed your action plan. Perhaps you need to try another solution to completely solve the problem. What could you do differently? Use the Reviewing Your Progress form on the facing page to evaluate your action plan.

Remember also that some stress-related problems just can't be solved by changing the situation. Think back to the ABC model of stress (from Chapter 3). Problem-solving techniques aim to change the A's—stressful events themselves. But sometimes this can't be done, or it works temporarily but is not a long-term fix. If you're having difficulties solving a problem using the techniques in this chapter, it might mean that you'll need to work on changing your B's—your beliefs and thoughts—about the problem. In Chapter 8 you'll learn how to change the kinds of B's that cause stress.

Regardless of your results, by working through this chapter you've learned and/or improved important new skills for how to deal with problems and work out solutions. Take some time to recognize how hard you've worked. And give yourself a pat on the back because this is an important part of stress management. If you've made it this far, it means that you're off to a great start. Keep practicing!

REVIEWING YOUR PROGRESS

1. What was the result of your action plan? Describe how well it worked.

2. What is the status of the problem? How close is it to being solved?

3. What obstacles came up that were not expected?

4. What could you have done differently to make the solution more effective?

5. What's the next step in resolving this problem (or what's the next problem to work on)?

6

Communicating Effectively

It's a fact: how you interact with other people—whether or not they're important in your life—influences your stress level. Do you have trouble saying no or standing up for yourself? Do you feel like others take advantage of you too easily? It might be that you don't communicate assertively enough. Do you have trouble with friendships, romantic partnerships, or getting along with people at work, school, or in everyday interactions? Polishing up your communication skills can help reduce these sources of stress too. It's a vicious cycle. As the diagram below shows, ineffective communication leads to relationship problems, which lead to stress. And when you're stressed out, it's more difficult to communicate effectively and assertively, so the relationship problems persist. In this chapter you'll see your way out of the vicious cycle by learning to how to effectively express your own needs and how to sidestep being easily manipulated by others. You'll also receive some tips for honing your listening and speaking skills so you can increase your enjoyment—and decrease your stress—in your relationships with others.

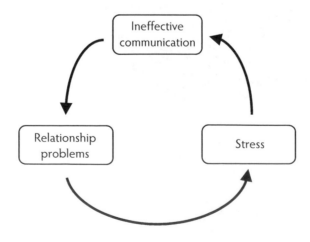

BUILDING ASSERTIVENESS SKILLS

Imagine yourself in the following situations. Describe how you'd normally react:

1. You've lent some money to a friend, but you wonder whether he forgot that he needs to repay you. What would you do?

_____

_____

2. At a restaurant you order a regular hamburger but get a cheeseburger—and you don't like cheese. What would you do?

_____

_____

3. The babysitter you hired to watch the kids tonight calls at the last minute to say that her best friend needs a ride to the airport, and she's going to be 2 hours late, ruining your plans for dinner and a movie. What would you do?

_____

_____

4. You have ticket #33 at the bakery, but after the person with #32 is finished, someone else without a ticket steps up to the counter and starts to place an order. What would you do?

_____

_____

5. Aunt Edna, with whom you prefer not to spend much time, is on the phone. She's just told you of her plans to spend 3 weeks visiting you, beginning next week. What would you do?

_____

_____

We'll return to use these scenarios later in the chapter. For now, know that how you would handle similar situations indicates your ability to be assertive. Assertiveness is a style of communicating in which you feel comfortable:

- Expressing your likes, dislikes, interests, opinions, and feelings

- Disagreeing with others, saying no, and taking a stand

- Asking others for favors

- Accepting (and giving) compliments and talking about yourself

- Asking for clarification

Assertive communication reduces conflict. It leads to better self-esteem and strong, supportive relationships involving mutual respect. How does it do that? Because when you act assertively, you not only stand up for yourself and act in your own best interests, expressing your feelings honestly and comfortably; you do so without violating the rights of others. No wonder research shows that people who behave more assertively have less stress in their lives: there's a difference between being assertive and being either aggressive or passive.

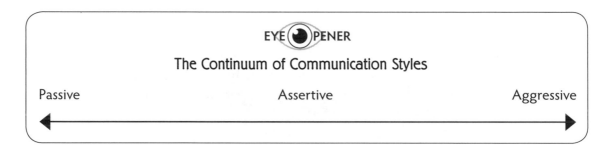

Aggressive, Passive, and Assertive Styles

Assertive communication falls in the middle of a continuum ranging from passive (non-assertive) to aggressive. All three styles have their advantages and disadvantages, although assertiveness is clearly the most advantageous. As you read on, keep the following scenario in mind: imagine that you're at a movie theater and the person sitting next to you keeps talking during the movie. It's disruptive and you're feeling annoyed.

Passive Communication

Passive communication means denying your own needs and holding back your real feelings. If you were to sit there in silence in the movie theater, deciding that the other person had the right to talk and be disruptive, you'd gain the advantage of not ruffling anyone's feathers. Being passive means keeping people on your "good side." But this benefit comes at a cost. Inside, you'll feel frustrated over not expressing how you really feel. You'd be

__People__ aren't "passive," "aggressive," "passive–aggressive," or "assertive." These are simply different styles of __communication__. In fact, most people use all of these styles at one time or another. The more you practice assertiveness, though, the more you'll be using a style that reduces stress.

living at the whim of others, not getting what you really want. You'd be easy to manipulate and take advantage of. Holding back your frustrations, of course, only increases your stress because you're still subject to the problem that caused you stress in the first place. And now it's probably bubbling away in your mind, growing bigger every minute.

Aggressive Communication

The opposite of the passive style is the *aggressive* style. When you get angry, attack others verbally (or physically), raise your voice, use sarcasm, or boss and bully others into giving you what you want, you're acting aggressively. For example, if in the movie theater you yelled, "You'd better stop talking, you moron, or I'll kick your @$$!" you'd certainly be heard, and you might get what you want (by bullying). But if this was your style, you'd also scare people away and end up without many friends. People with anger problems often have very stressful lives. And it's this type of anger and hostility that's linked with stress-related medical problems like heart attacks and strokes.

EYE PENER

Passive–Aggressive Communication

There's also a *passive–aggressive* style of communication in which you express yourself indirectly and often in ways that are not very nice or effective in getting what you want. For example, instead of actually saying something to the person talking in the movie theater, you let him know you're bothered by sighing loudly.

Assertive Communication

The *assertive* communication style takes the best of both worlds. You make sure that other people know your feelings and desires, but you do this in an appropriate, courteous, and respectful (nonaggressive) way that doesn't offend or bully others. In the movie situation, an assertive response might be to firmly yet politely say, "Please stop talking. I'm having trouble hearing the movie. Thank you." The main advantage of assertive behavior is that you're standing up for yourself without being rude or bossy. The main disadvantage is that you might not always get what you want. But at least you won't feel guilty or taken advantage of—you'll have spoken up for yourself. There is, however, more to assertiveness than dealing with difficult people and situations. Being assertive means feeling secure about expressing positive feelings toward others—love, intimacy, admiration, appreciation. It means being gracious about accepting compliments and thanks. When you feel good about how you deal with all of these situations, you feel less stressed. With assertive communication, the pros far outweigh the cons.

How to Think Assertively

Before you're ready to *behave* assertively, you need to be able to *think* assertively. That's right, assertiveness is as much a frame of mind as it is a set of skills. Research shows that people who act more assertively believe that, like everyone else, they have a right to their own feelings, beliefs, and opinions—including the right to express them. They also believe all humans are equal and meant to treat each other as equals. They're secure in their own experiences and don't need others to tell them how to think or feel. In short, they're not hung up on making sure they have everyone's approval all the time.

> *People who act assertively realize that you can't please everyone all the time. They don't need others' approval for their own thoughts, beliefs, and feelings.*

The *Assertiveness Bill of Rights* in the box below contains a list of rights that people who act assertively believe all human beings are entitled to. Do you feel you're entitled to these rights? If not, your ideas about relationships and communication might be colored by overly rigid views and beliefs such as those listed here and on the top of the facing page:

- "I'm not as good or important as other people."

- "I should never put my own needs ahead of others."

- "I should be perfect . . . *always*."

Assertiveness Bill of Rights

All human beings have the right to what's listed below. I'm entitled to these things every bit as much as everyone else.

- Expressing my own feelings and opinions
- Asking for help and emotional support
- Saying no and disputing unfair treatment
- Making mistakes
- Disagreeing with anyone (even authority figures)
- Changing my mind
- Not having to justify myself to others
- Ignoring the advice of others if I choose

- "I shouldn't waste others' time talking about my successes or problems."

- "I'm never entitled to question what others tell or teach me."

- "I must have others' approval."

But all of these beliefs and ideas are false. They're rigid and exaggerated. What's more, they'll stifle your efforts at becoming more assertive and keep you from reducing stress. Here's an exercise to help you avoid these thinking traps and get into the assertive state of mind:

1. First, describe a recent situation with another person—an argument, making a decision, or the like—when you wished you'd acted more assertively. What did you say? What was your tone of voice? How did you hold yourself? How much eye contact did you make?

   _____

   _____

2. Then try to remember what you were thinking and feeling just before and during the situation. Write down what was running through your head. What were you telling yourself? (*Hint: The theme probably had something to do with your ideas or wishes not being as important as the other person's—perhaps one of the beliefs in the bulleted list you just read.*)

   _____

   _____

3. Next, think about how you could have changed what you were thinking in #2. What could you have told yourself about the other person or the situation that would have helped you be more assertive? (*Hint: Try something from the Assertiveness Bill of Rights on the facing page.*)

   _____

   _____

4. If you were thinking these new thoughts, how would you feel? How would your behavior be different? What sort of language would you use? What would your tone of voice sound like? How would you be holding yourself? How much eye contact would you make?

   _____

   _____

EYE OPENER

Assertive Beliefs

The beliefs in the bulleted list that runs from page 106 to page 107 are maladaptive and exaggerated. They're illogical and dysfunctional, and they lead to unassertive behavior. Here are logical alternatives that will lead to acting more assertively:

- "I'm just as good as everyone else. My feelings matter just as much as anyone else's."

- "I have the right to put my own needs ahead of others' without explaining myself."

- "I can't be perfect—to err is human. Everyone makes mistakes, and that's okay."

- "I have the right to talk about my feelings, successes, and problems with others."

- "I have the right to use my brain to think about and question whatever I want."

- "Although it can be nice to have, I don't need others' approval to do or think as I wish."

How to Act Assertively

I Statements

"*I* statements" are the building blocks of assertive communication because you're speaking for yourself and remaining objective. They're the best way to let other people know you're upset about something without making accusations or putting the other person down. That's because in *I* statements you don't directly link your displeasure with the other person's behavior. And this maintains a good relationship between you and the listener. Some examples of *I* statements for different situations appear in the table on facing page.

> *I statements help you manage stress because you can tell others how you feel without directly accusing them or making them feel bad.*

In any situation, there's no one "best" *I* statement. In fact, you might be able to think of different (or better) ones for the scenarios shown in the table. Here are the main things to keep in mind when coming up with them:

- Acknowledge only the facts of the situation—what you can observe with your five senses. This does *not* include your perception of other people's motives or intentions.

- Acknowledge that how *you* feel about the situation is your own point of view and not necessarily how everyone else sees it.

- State your viewpoint in a way that doesn't blame or put down other people—even if they really *are* to blame. It might be tempting to finger-point, but this will only make others defensive and increase everyone's stress.

I statements are such an important part of assertiveness that it's worth spending the time to practice them. So, next to each of the situations that follow, try writing your own *I* statement response. As you work through this chapter, you'll see more about how to use *I* statements.

1. At work, you're asked to be on a committee that you don't want to be on:

_____

_____

2. The cashier at the store gives you back too little change:

_____

_____

Typical *I* Statements

Situation	Example	*I* statement
You need to confront someone about his behavior	You find out a coworker is talking about you behind your back	"I don't like it when people say things about me behind my back. My feelings are hurt and I'm asking you to stop."
You feel someone is treating you wrong or being unfair	Your roommate or partner doesn't help with chores	"I don't like when we leave the trashcan full because the apartment starts to smell bad."
You feel angry	Your mother just revealed to a friend something about your private life that you wanted to keep private	"Mother, that's something very private that I didn't want out in the open. I'm feeling very angry and embarrassed right now."
Someone is angry with you	You accidentally rear-ended another driver at a stoplight, and now she's telling you off	"I rear-ended your car, and I'm very sorry. It was an accident, but I understand why you're very angry."

3. Someone you thought was your friend gets you in trouble at work:

_____

_____

4. You're trying to study in the library, and someone is being very loud:

_____

_____

5. Your neighbor's dog is using your front lawn for his bathroom:

_____

_____

Assertive Problem Solving

Once you've got the hang of _I_ statements, communicating assertively requires relatively few steps. The first step is to think about the various situations in your life where using a more assertive style could be helpful—dealing with a relative, a coworker, a boss, or a peer group; returning something you bought back to the store; giving or accepting compliments. Take some time to consider several situations in which you would like to be more assertive and list these below:

I would like to be more assertive when . . .

1. _____

2. _____

3. _____

4. _____

5. _____

6. _____

7. _____

You'll probably use assertiveness skills most often to deal with situations in which there is some sort of disagreement or problem that needs to be worked out between you and someone else (or a group). Do any of the situations you wrote down fit into this category? If so, choose one to develop a sample _assertive script_ for what to do and say. If not, think of how you might apply what you read in this section the next time such an issue pops up. The acronym DEAR provides a helpful way to remember the basics of assertive problem solving:

D *Define* **the problem**. Explain the issue to the other person. But make sure you stick to objective facts rather than opinions or finger-pointing. Simply state what happened and what the problem is. For example, "I brought my car in on Monday and was told that it would be fixed and ready for me by Friday at 5:00. Now it's Friday and you're saying it won't be ready until next week sometime. I'm wondering how we can solve this problem."

E *Express* **your feelings**. Use *I* statements to let the other person know how you feel without finger-pointing or directly blaming him. Try to word this so that the other person can relate to what you're going through. For example, "I'm feeling frustrated because I was counting on being able to take the car on a trip for my job this weekend. I'm sure you understand." Make sure you don't substitute an *opinion* for a *feeling* ("I feel that your repair shop stinks!"). In other words, don't use *you* statements disguised as *I* statements. You'll only put the other person on the defensive and lose any chance of getting what you want.

A *Ask* **for what you want.** You can't expect others to read your mind. So, in a fair, concise, and firm way, tell the other person your wish. But rather than assuming that you're entitled to get what you want (which is *not* one of your rights as a human being), state this as a *preference*, not a *command*. For example, "I'd like to pick up my car on Friday at 5:00 or if it's not ready, get a rental car from you so I can go on my trip."

R **Provide** *reinforcement.* End by letting the other person know that you appreciate her help. The best way is to describe the positive consequences of accommodating your wish. For example, "Thanks for understanding. I appreciate your help. Next time I need a repair, I'll feel good about bringing my car back to your shop."

Sometimes positive reinforcement doesn't work. If you're having trouble motivating the other person to find ways to help you, it might be worth mentioning some *negative* consequences—that is, how you'll stand up for yourself if you don't get what you're asking for. I'm not talking about making threats—that will just anger the other person and do more harm than good. Rather, simply state the consequences of noncooperation and be sure you're willing to back it up. For example, "If my car won't be ready by 5:00 as promised, and you're not willing to lend me a car for the weekend, then just leave my car alone. I'll pick it up and take my business elsewhere."

Now it's time for you to practice assertiveness. Start by using the Assertive Response worksheet on the next page to come up with a response to one of the situations you listed on page 110. Make copies of this form so you can use it to formulate other assertive responses too. Page 113 shows an example that was completed by Mindy, who was asked to host a retirement party for a colleague and was feeling uncomfortable about saying no to her supervisor.

ASSERTIVE RESPONSE

Define the problem. In very specific, objective terms, describe the situation you're concerned about.

Express your feelings using *I* statements. How do you feel about the situation?

Ask for what you want. Describe your wishes for resolving the situation. How would you like things to change?

Reinforcement. How will the other person be rewarded for giving you what you want? What's in it for him or her?

Using the information above, write a concise script that follows the DEAR format that you can use when talking to the other person:

Just in case, what are some possible negative consequences for the other person if your wishes are not accommodated?

ASSERTIVE RESPONSE: MINDY

Define the problem. In very specific, objective terms, describe the situation you're concerned about:

My supervisor at work, Elizabeth, asked me to throw a retirement party for Linda, who is retiring next month. I don't really want to do this because it will take up lots of time and I'm already busy with work and being a single parent. Plus, I'll end up spending a lot of money that I won't get back. However, I already said yes.

Express your feelings using *I* statements. How do you feel about the situation?

I'm feeling overwhelmed with work and with being the single parent of two school-age kids. Having to plan a retirement party is the last thing I need to be doing.

Ask for what you want. Describe your wishes for resolving the situation. How would you like things to change?

I'd like for someone else to take the lead in planning this party. At the very least, I'd like to have a co-planner who will take some of the load off my shoulders.

Reinforcement. How will the other person be rewarded for giving you what you want? What's in it for him or her?

It would be a better party if someone else planned it or if someone helped me.

Using the information above, write a concise script that follows the DEAR format that you can use when talking to the other person:

Elizabeth, I wanted to talk to you about Linda's retirement party. I know I agreed to plan it, but I'm really feeling overwhelmed right now between my work projects and my kids needing my attention. I feel I made a mistake when I said I'd plan the party the other day; I'd actually prefer not to be in charge of it after all. I'm sorry for changing my mind. I hope you understand.

Just in case, what are some possible negative consequences for the other person if your wishes are not accommodated?

I would say that I'm afraid Linda might not be happy with her retirement party if I'm left in charge.

Resolving Conflicts and Avoiding Manipulation

Just because you communicate assertively doesn't mean you're guaranteed to get what you want out of the situation. The other person might have his or her own reasons for not accommodating you (as the song goes, *you can't always get what you want*). The *passive* response here is to just give in and go along with the other person. The *aggressive* response would be anger. But as you've learned, these approaches increase your stress.

Instead, here are some *assertive* strategies for trying to resolve standoffs and conflicts in your favor. They'll also help you sidestep attempts to manipulate you by others. The advantages of these techniques: you know you've stuck up for yourself, tried your best, and probably garnered some respect from the other person. The disadvantage: you're *still* not guaranteed to get your way.

Broken Record Technique

This involves respectfully but firmly restating your point each time someone denies your assertive request. If the other person gets angry or brings up other (past) issues, acknowledge that you've heard what she said, but resist discussing these and become a broken record. Here's an example relating to Mindy's situation with the retirement party.

ELIZABETH: The other day you agreed to this, Mindy.

MINDY: I realize that, but I've decided that I'd prefer not to be in charge of planning the retirement party.

ELIZABETH: You'll find the time to do it. I'm sure you'll do a good job.

MINDY: I appreciate that, but I'd prefer not to be in charge of planning the retirement party.

ELIZABETH: You know, it's not good to go back on your word.

MINDY: I realize I'm changing my mind, but I'd prefer not to be in charge of planning the retirement party.

ELIZABETH: This isn't the first time you've changed your mind once you agreed to something. Do you remember the situation with the parking passes a few months ago?

MINDY: I do remember that, but as I've said, I'd really prefer not to be in charge of planning the retirement party.

Turning the Tables

When a standstill is reached in your conversation, it's an assertive move to point this out. Then ask the other person how he thinks the problem should be resolved. For example, Mindy might say to Elizabeth, "It looks like we're going around in circles here. I originally agreed to plan the party, but changed my mind after giving it some thought. How can we get past this?" When you try turning the tables, you might just get a compromise you can live with. But be prepared to continue your assertive role if the other person suggests something you don't wish to go along with.

Time-Outs

If you sense the other person becoming angry, an assertive move is to refuse to continue the discussion. Instead, take a "time-out" until she has calmed down. You might say, "I can see you're very upset right now. Let's continue this discussion later this afternoon." Use the same strategy if you feel yourself becoming angry. You don't want to become overly emotional, because it's harder for you to think clearly and maintain your assertive stance. Try saying something like "I understand what you're saying, but I need some time to think it over" or "I'm not ready to talk about this right now. Let me find you in a little while."

Pointing Out the Process or the Emotion

Some people might respond to your assertiveness by trying to change the subject. For example, you're letting someone know how you feel about her behavior, and rather than listen, she (unassertively) raises a separate issue (such as dredging up something from the past) or attacks you personally (like calling you a name). When this occurs, the best course of action is to point out what's happening in the conversation (that is, the *process*) and bring it back to what you wanted to discuss. For instance, "I see that we're getting off the topic. We were talking about _____" or "These are old issues between us, and we can talk about them another time. Right now, we're discussing _____." If the person becomes quiet or teary-eyed (another form of manipulation), point this out as well: "I can see that this is hard for you to talk about. I wonder what's making you feel uncomfortable." This strategy also works if the person responds to your assertiveness by trying to make a joke ("Jokes are getting us off the topic. We're talking about _____ right now") or by splitting hairs with you about whether your thoughts and feelings are legitimate ("That's not really the point. We've gotten off the topic . . . ").

Agreement with a Twist

When someone criticizes you (for example, "You really messed up this time"), an assertive response is to simply agree and find some way to credit the critic or use just a bit of self-effacing humor (this is the "twist" part). For example, "Yeah, I really bombed *this time*, didn't I? I appreciate your pointing it out—as if it was hard to notice!" This defuses the critic—you've acknowledged the criticism (about this particular time) and even one-upped it! But whatever happens, don't get defensive or feel like you need to save face. That will only give the critic more ammunition. Remember that no one is perfect (even your critic!)—you're entitled to mess up. Also, remember that you don't owe anyone an explanation if you don't want to give one. Finally, don't make any promises about doing better next time—this only opens the door to more criticism and makes you look passive.

Let's say someone puts you down *as a person* because of something you did ("You didn't complete the project correctly. You can't do anything right! You're just an idiot"). Here, agree in part: try to find something constructive you can see eye to eye on . . . but ignore the hostile personal remarks. For example, "Yes, you're right. I sure botched *this one*."

Assertive Questioning

Another assertive strategy for avoiding being manipulated by someone else's anger or personal attack is to ask specific questions about it. For example, ask the person to clarify what she doesn't like, as in the following dialogue:

> YOU: I can tell you're upset with me. What is it about my behavior that's bothering you?
>
> SOMEONE ELSE: You're just socially inept.
>
> YOU: What about me do you feel is socially inept?
>
> SOMEONE ELSE: You say the wrong things at the wrong time.
>
> YOU: Okay. I'm sure I've done that *sometimes*. What about that bothers you so much?"

This strategy also works if someone responds to your assertiveness with a threat, such as "If you keep nagging me, I'm going to call Human Resources." To this, you could point out the process and use assertive questioning: "That sounds like a threat. We're just having a discussion. What specifically am I saying or doing that you don't like?" Notice that these questions focus the discussion on *behaviors* and ignore the personal attacks or threats.

Know Your Limit

Have an idea of how far you're willing to bend and go along with the other person. If your standoff continues despite using these other tactics, perhaps you'll make a concession. Mindy, for example, knew that she could manage to plan the retirement party if she had a co-planner. So, if she and Elizabeth got into a stalemate, she could suggest a co-planner as a last resort. For example, "I guess you're not going to change your mind about this. So, I'd like to find someone to be my co-planner. This would relieve me of half the work, and I'd feel a lot better about giving Linda the kind of retirement party she deserves." Remember to use reinforcement strategies when suggesting any alternatives. This creates a "win-win situation" in which both parties feel like they're getting something out of the compromise.

Giving Compliments and Criticism Assertively

Compliments

Expressing your positive feelings by complimenting others can be a very rewarding experience. You'll make someone else feel good—maybe even brighten her day—and her positive feedback (such as a "thank you" or smile) will in turn make you feel good. It's assertive to let people know when you feel good about something they've done. Soon they'll be giving you compliments too. Talk about reducing interpersonal stress! Here are some tips for giving compliments:

- **Be specific.** Point out a particular behavior to compliment the other person on (and use *I* statements). So, rather than saying "You did a good job in that meeting," say something like "I was really impressed with how you ran that meeting, especially how you listened to everyone's points and made some good suggestions." Try to let the other person know how you feel about what he or she did.

- **Praise *behaviors*, not *people*.** Remember the problem with labels? It's not *people* that are good or bad, it's their *behaviors* (people can't be distilled down to adjectives, but actions can be). We all do good and bad things. So, when giving compliments, praise *what* the person did ("George, you did a great job with the Penske file!"), not *who* he is ("George, you're great guy!").

- **Give reasons for your compliments.** People like to know why they're being praised. For example, "I'm very proud of the way you finished your homework today. Rather than put it off until after dinner, you came home and got right to work. Great job."

- **Don't overdo it.** Compliment others in moderation. If you're always dishing out large portions of praise, it will come to mean less and less, and people may even get tired of hearing it. Also, make sure your compliments fit the achievement. That is, make sure the amount of praise you give, and how you give it, is appropriate. Some achievements (such as winning a marathon or getting into a good college) are worth getting very excited about, while others (such as running a smooth meeting or choosing a nice restaurant) deserve a more measured response.

- **Smile and speak up.** As you'll read more about later, others pick up on your body language. Make sure the message you send with your body fits your words. Look the person in the eye, smile, and confidently give your compliment. You'll seem more genuine.

Now it's time to give it a try. In the spaces below, write out a compliment for each situation:

1. Your coworker, Marla, just got a promotion: _____
   _____

2. Your kids raved about Samantha, the babysitter they had last night. You want to call her and let her know: _____
   _____

3. Your English professor, Dr. Jackson, published a book that you read and enjoyed: _____

4. A neighbor you haven't seen in a while has lost a lot of weight: _____

5. You were impressed by the sermon you heard at your place of worship. Afterwards, you run into the person who gave the sermon: _____

EYE OPENER

Accepting Compliments

Do you have trouble accepting compliments? A lot of people do—it can be awkward. And there's an assertive and an unassertive way to accept them. Some people become nervous or bashful when they're complimented. Others object or downplay their accomplishment. But this is passive behavior that makes you seem less confident and makes the other person uncomfortable. Here are some *dos* and *don'ts* when someone pays you a compliment:

Do:

Smile! The person giving you the compliment wants you to feel good. So don't let her down or she won't be so quick to praise you again. Remember that you're just as entitled to compliments as anyone else. Smile when you receive a compliment—be proud of yourself. Look the person in the eye and . . .

Give thanks. A simple and graceful "Thank you, I appreciate that" or "Thanks, that means a lot to me" is all you really need to say. It's not hard, and it will help you feel more confident. And no, you don't need to pay the person back with a compliment of your own.

Practice. In the mirror. Imagine someone has just said something nice to you. Then say something like "Aww, thank you. That's so nice of you to say."

Don't:

Object. The person complimenting you is going out of his way to make you feel good. The last thing you want to do is insult him by disagreeing ("Oh no, I was awful").

Explain yourself. You don't need to explain or make excuses for doing something well! Refrain from saying things like "Thanks, I worked really hard at it" or "It cost a lot." These can seem rude or egotistical.

Shy away. Don't change the topic of conversation without acknowledging the compliment. The other person was being genuine, and you should return the favor. You might even use the compliment to focus the conversation on something you can both talk about. For example, "Thanks, I had a terrific guitar teacher. You know, he once played on tour with the Grateful Dead."

The best way to get comfortable giving compliments is to practice. At least once a day (but only if it's genuine and appropriate), push yourself to give someone a compliment. It's a low-risk action (most people will give you positive feedback), and soon enough you'll be feeling confident about doing this more often.

Assertive Body Language

Did you know that in face-to-face encounters with other people, 93% of your communication is with your *body*? Words make up only 7% of communication. That means *body language*—the unspoken (nonverbal) communication that we all use in everyday face-to-face meetings—is even more powerful than anything you say out loud. Which is why learning assertive body language is so important. Just like your words, body language influences how people treat you. It can make the difference between getting what you want and being taken advantage of. Because of this, using assertive body language can help reduce your stress levels. This section contains some tips and suggestions for using assertive, stress-reducing body language.

Eye Contact

Make this a priority—it's probably the most important nonverbal way to communicate. Looking a person in the eye is assertive because it shows that you're confident and respectful. But remember, it's not a staring contest! Don't glare—this will make the other person uncomfortable. Remain relaxed and occasionally look away. Also keep in mind that looking down too much suggests you're not sure of yourself. It sends the signal that you can be taken advantage of.

Shaking Hands

A firm (but not overpowering) handshake signals confidence and security. You're more likely to be taken seriously than if your hand feels like a dead fish when someone shakes it.

Posture, Distance, and Angling

Stand up straight when you need to be assertive. Shoulders back and stomach sucked in. You'll feel taller and stronger and more confident than if you're slouching forward. Hold your head up to show self-assurance. This tells the other person, "What I'm saying is important."

Don't stand too close to the other person, as this may be seen as a sign of aggression. On the other hand, standing too far away makes you appear distant or shy. Finally, angle your body toward the person you're speaking to. He'll take this as a sign that you're interested in him. If you're angled away, he's sure to think you distrust him or don't like him.

Don't fold your arms across your chest. This unassertive posture gives the signal that you're defensive and not open to communicating. Use arm and hand gestures to emphasize the importance of your ideas and messages. But don't talk too much with your hands; it's a sign of nervousness. And too much (and very strong) hand gesturing can be a sign of aggression.

Facial Expressions

Make sure your expression is consistent with what you're saying and how you're feeling. If you're giving a compliment, smile. If you're upset, don't. Your face should be sending the same message as your words.

Your Tone of Voice

Although it's not exactly a part of body language, your tone influences how people listening to you receive what you're saying. When you speak in a deliberate way using a quiet tone and lower (deeper) pitch, you come across as more in control and self-confident and your words are taken more seriously than if you speak in a higher, louder voice, which suggests that you're tense, anxious, and unsure of yourself.

Now it's time to put it all together and practice your assertiveness skills. Remember the situations you responded to on page 103? Try to imagine yourself in them one more

---

EYE PENER

Tips for Becoming More Assertive

Using assertive communication is a skill, and like any other skill, it requires time and practice (lots of practice). Here are some suggestions:

1. **Watch others.** Keep a lookout for when others act assertively—especially people you admire. Make a mental note of how they approach the situation. What do they say, and how do they say it? How do they think about the situation (you might interview them to find out)?

2. **Easy does it.** Use a gradual approach. To get your feet wet with assertiveness skills, try them out first in easy situations. Then, when you're feeling more comfortable, challenge yourself to try them under more and more difficult circumstances.

3. **Keep a diary.** Try keeping an assertiveness diary (like the one on page 122). Monitoring your behavior is a great way to motivate yourself to work harder.

4. **Don't beat yourself up.** When you're not successful using assertiveness skills—and this happens to just about everyone at some point—don't get down on yourself. Instead, use it as a learning experience and analyze the situation. What should you do differently next time?

time. But now use what you know about assertive communication to come up with assertive reactions:

1. You've lent some money to a friend, but you wonder whether he forgot that he needs to repay you. What would you do? _____

    _____

    _____

2. At a restaurant you order a regular hamburger but get a cheeseburger—and you don't like cheese. What would you do? _____

    _____

    _____

3. The babysitter you hired to watch the kids tonight calls at the last minute to say that her best friend needs a ride to the airport, and she's going to be 2 hours late, ruining your plans for dinner and a movie. What would you do? _____

    _____

    _____

4. You have ticket #33 at the bakery, but after the person with #32 is finished, someone else steps up to the counter and starts to place an order. What would you do? _____

    _____

    _____

5. Aunt Edna, with whom you prefer not to spend much time, is on the phone. She's just told you of her plans to spend 3 weeks visiting you, beginning next week. What would you do? _____

    _____

    _____

On the next page is an assertiveness diary. You can use it to keep track of when you use assertive behavior and when you don't. Remember that keeping track of your actions (or *self-monitoring*) is one of the best ways to change your behavior. Self-monitoring keeps you accountable—you have a record of how well you're doing with using certain skills so you can see how you're progressing. This particular diary will also help you detect any patterns in your assertive or nonassertive behavior. For instance, do you have trouble acting assertively with certain people or in certain situations? Finally, keeping an honest diary of your assertiveness will help you track changes over time. It's my hope that, as you practice more and more, you'll use these skills more often and they'll bring better and better results.

ASSERTIVENESS DIARY

Complete this form whenever you're in a situation that calls for assertiveness. In the first column, enter the date and time. Next, briefly describe the situation. In the third column, enter the names of any key people involved in the situation. Then check whether you handled the situation assertively or not and describe what you did. Finally, briefly note what you might have done to handle the situation even better or more assertively. The first row contains an example you can follow.

Date/time	Situation (brief description)	Key people involved	What I did		Thoughts about how I handled the situation
June 11 3:15 pm	A child and her mother showed up at the door selling Girl Scout cookies, and I didn't want to buy any.	Girl Scout and her mother—I didn't know them	☑ Assertive I said "No thanks. We already have plenty of cookies in the house."	☐ Unassertive	I did a good job saying no, but I didn't have to give an explanation.
			☐ Assertive	☐ Unassertive	
			☐ Assertive	☐ Unassertive	
			☐ Assertive	☐ Unassertive	
			☐ Assertive	☐ Unassertive	

ANTI-STRESS LISTENING

You've probably never thought much about what it really means to listen to someone, and most of us wouldn't believe our own listening skills have much to do with our stress levels. But think about it: When you leave your boss's or your doctor's office after receiving a list of instructions and then go back to your cubicle or home and realize you have only a partial picture of what you're supposed to do, what happens? Your stress goes up as you imagine doing something that will compromise your health or your job status. Let's say your wife is complaining that you don't spend enough time with the family and then suddenly blows up, accusing you of having one foot out the door and "clearly not listening to a word" she says. You resent the assumption and wonder how your relationship could be so shaky these days. Listening is a lot more powerful than most of us believe; and much more complicated. Here are some tips and reminders about aspects of listening that affect stress the most.

Does Stress Get in the Way of Paying Attention When Others Are Speaking to You?

When you're stressed, your mind might be going a million miles an hour in all different directions. But often the person speaking to you is all too aware that your focus has drifted away. Staying focused on the speaker (even if you think you know what she is going to say) helps you hear better and lets the speaker know you're tuned in—right away you've headed off potential conflict and stress in this particular interaction.

Here are some *dos* and *don'ts* to keep in mind for listening attentively:

- Don't look around the room or out the window.
- Never check your watch, phone, or e-mail in the middle of a conversation.
- If the surroundings are distracting, ask to continue the conversation in a quieter place.
- If you receive a phone call, politely ask if it's okay if you see who is calling, but answer only calls that absolutely can't wait. If you receive a text message, wait until the conversation is over to read or respond to it. Pretend there will be a test on what the speaker is saying!
- Listen for "take-home messages." The main ideas the speaker wants to get across to you might come at the start or end of a talk and often get repeated.
- If you're not sure you understand what someone has said, just ask for clarification.

Does Stress Keep You from Being an Active Listener?

Passive listening—being a receptacle rather than a participant—usually robs you of the speaker's full message and doesn't cultivate good relationships. Active listening involves using verbal and nonverbal strategies that help you hear and understand more fully and foster a connection between you and the speaker, encouraging him to share more information. Here are some *dos* and *don'ts* for active listening:

- Respond with an occasional "I see" or "Oh really?" at appropriate times.

- You can also wait for the speaker to pause and then paraphrase what she has just said using your own words. For example:

  SPEAKER: I have three kids in grade school. They're involved in lots of different after-school activities—piano, baseball, dance. Just getting them to their activities and watching their recitals and games is like a full-time job.

  YOU: Wow, sounds like they keep you pretty busy.

- Comment on bits of information you hear. For example:

  SPEAKER: My wife's been in the hospital all week. She suddenly became very ill on Monday, and I've had to take care of the kids while she's in there.

  YOU: Geez. I'm sorry to hear that. It must be hard for you to manage things around the house without her help.

- This type of response not only shows the other person that you're listening; it demonstrates that you can relate to what he is saying. Look directly at the speaker, sitting up straight (perhaps leaning toward him) and making appropriate eye contact.

- Unfold your arms and legs as a sign of openness, and nod now and then to show that you understand what's being said.

- Using appropriate facial expressions—a smile, frown, look of surprise, or a raised eyebrow—also lets the speaker know that you're interested.

Do You Get the Urge to Interrupt When People Are Talking to You?

It can be hard not to interrupt if you're under a lot of stress, feel the pressure to move conversations along and get on with everything else on your plate. But we all appreciate having the chance to say everything we'd like to without being interrupted, and relationships are weakened when one party feels denied that opportunity. Here are some *dos* and *don'ts* for resisting interrupting:

- Let the speaker finish before you start talking. In other words, take turns speaking. Resist the urge to finish people's sentences for them. Interjecting sends the message that you're not listening—even when you really are.

- Try not to think too much about how to make a brilliant comeback while the speaker is still talking. It seems natural to start thinking about what you're going to say—a convincing debate point, witty wisecrack, or better story—before the other person is finished speaking; but while you're mentally rehearsing your retort you're not listening to what the other person is saying.

How to Practice Anti-Stress Listening

It may seem strange to practice something you've been doing all your life. But as with any other skill, you'll only become more effective at listening (and enhance your relationships) when you work at it:

- Think of someone who you have a hard time listening to and practice using the skills in this section to listen very carefully to that person each time you speak with him or her.

- Put on that talk radio station you never listen to. If you're a liberal, listen to a conservative talk show. If you hate sports, listen to a sports talk show. Forcing yourself to listen and pay attention to something you disagree with, or a topic you're just not that interested in, is an excellent way to hone your listening skills.

- What do you find boring? A coworker who drones on and on at meetings? A lecture about butterflies or saving the environment? A golf telecast? Whatever it is, seek it out and force yourself to listen. Pay attention to what's being said. You might not enjoy the exercise, but with practice you'll get better at listening.

ANTI-STRESS SPEAKING

As with listening, there are many ways that stress can shape how we speak and end up making a bad situation worse. The following are four of the most common, with *dos* and *don'ts* for keeping stress from affecting your speaking style and for de-escalating stress while speaking.

Do You Feel Like You Have to Get Involved in Tough Discussions Even Though You're Stressed?

Sometimes just letting people know how you feel takes some of the edge off. Before you say something you'll regret, warn those around you of how you're feeling. Let them know you're in a lousy mood or under a lot of pressure. Tell them this might not be the best time to have a serious conversation. If it's too late and you've already said some unpleasant things (or used a nasty tone of voice), own up to your mistake. Give a genuine apology for your outburst and say that you feel bad and will try your best not to let it happen again.

Do You Use *You* or *Global* Statements Instead of *I* Statements?

When we're already under stress and something happens that makes us feel even worse, a common reflex is to strike out and blame someone else for the problem: "*You* picked a terrible movie for us to see. I thought you had better taste!" Obviously, this is likely to put the other person on the defensive and increases the chances that he will respond in ways that escalate stress levels: "Screw you! It was a great movie. You're clueless."

Global statements are also common when you're stressed out and aren't much better: "This is the worst movie in the world. No one in his right mind could enjoy it!" When you make global statements, treating your own point of view as if it's a scientific fact, you're saying that the other person, who may very well have enjoyed the movie, is stupid or unsophisticated or otherwise beneath contempt. This is a sure path to escalating interpersonal stress, since the other person will feel compelled to prove you're wrong. Instead, use *I* statements as described on page 108. For example, "I really didn't care for that movie. I thought it was too predictable."

Do You Jump In to Offer Advice Too Quickly?

When you're under a lot of stress, you're constantly aware of having a lot of problems nagging at you to be solved. Being in this mode can make you assume that any issue brought up to you is a problem you're being asked to help solve. But sometimes the speaker may merely want to let you know how she's thinking or feeling about the issue. And however great and well-intentioned your ideas or solutions may be, the speaker in this situation will only be frustrated if you offer them. The result? Interpersonal conflict and more stress. Here are some *dos* and *don'ts* for avoiding giving unwanted advice:

- Don't offer advice unless the speaker asks for it.

- Listen carefully to find out what the other person wants from a conversation.

- If you don't know for sure what the speaker wants, there's no harm in asking: "Did you want to try to figure out a solution to this, or just discuss how you're feeling?"

- When the speaker just wants to talk about his feelings, use anti-stress listening skills to understand them. Show that you understand what he is saying—even if you don't completely agree—by summarizing his most important feelings, thoughts, or conflicts. For example, "So you're saying that you're angry because the neighbor keeps parking on the street in front of our house."

- Don't judge what the other person is saying or tell him that his feelings are wrong or irrational.

- Don't ask too many questions.

- Just be there for the other person. Make sure she feels listened to and understood. That's a good way to keep communication stress-free.

7

Time Management

"There's never enough time to do my work."

"There aren't enough hours in the day."

"I always end up cramming for exams."

"I didn't get anything productive done today."

"Where did all my free time go?"

"I'm always in a rush."

"Why do people always think I can fit one more thing into my schedule?"

Do you find yourself saying or thinking these types of things? If so, you probably know that feeling as if you always have too much to do and too little time to do it in can become a major source of stress. Maybe you chalk this up to the realities of modern life. Or you feel that it comes with the territory of being a person that others know they can count on. But it might also be that your time management skills could use a boost. That's what Alden discovered:

Alden, 42, manages a seaside resort hotel. He has lots of business but also lots of stress. Although Alden has hired extra staff to keep up with the growing workload, he generally subscribes to the belief "If you want something done right, you've got to do it yourself," and so he hasn't assigned his new workers a lot of jobs. As a result, he sometimes spends entire days doing menial tasks around the hotel; at other times he just stares out his office window, worrying about his ever-increasing to-do list, including the profit-producing tasks that would help him make his larger payroll. Even though he works long hours and weekends, Alden never seems to get enough done. Now his marriage is suffering—there's no time left to spend with his wife, kids, or friends. His daily jogging routine has also recently fallen by the wayside, not to mention his diet. Alden has gained weight. He spends late nights either at work or tossing and turning in bed, worried about everything he still has to do. Finally, he's developed daily headaches and fatigue from lack of sleep and realized what he's doing to himself.

Do you believe, as Alden does, that taking on more responsibilities will improve the outcome? In fact, it often does the opposite: taking on too many tasks can make anyone *less* productive overall and with individual tasks. When you take on more tasks than you can realistically do well, you become stressed and overwhelmed. You have less time to spend with each task, which makes you less effective. In the end, you might spend more time *worrying* about getting things done than it would take to actually *get* them done. And in their attempt to reduce their stress, some people try to tackle even more tasks— which just leads them into a vicious cycle. In this chapter, you'll learn techniques for managing your time better so you can get out of the vicious cycle.

HOW WELL DO YOU MANAGE YOUR TIME?

First, let's find out if this is a problem for you. Some people handle time pressures quite well. Others just don't know how to say no; if you believe this is the case for you, read Chapter 6, where you can polish your assertiveness skills. But also answer the following questions using the scale below to see if time management problems are an issue too:

	0 = Never	1 = Sometimes	2 = Always		
I complete tasks in order of priority.			0	1	2
I accomplish what I set out to do each day.			0	1	2
I get assignments done on time.			0	1	2
I feel I use my time effectively.			0	1	2
I complete difficult or unpleasant tasks without procrastinating.			0	1	2
I make time for planning my schedule.			0	1	2
I make daily or weekly to-do lists.			0	1	2
I meet deadlines without rushing at the last minute.			0	1	2
I prevent myself from being interrupted or distracted when working on high-priority tasks.			0	1	2
I avoid spending too much time on minor tasks.			0	1	2
I purposely plan time in my schedule to relax or be with friends.			0	1	2
I have a written or electronic schedule where I keep track of my commitments (meetings, classes, and so forth).			0	1	2

	0	1	2
I try to do the most important tasks during my most energetic periods of the day.	0	1	2
I make good use of my traveling time to be productive or relax.	0	1	2
I stop wasteful or unproductive activities and routines.	0	1	2
I screen my telephone calls to minimize interruptions.	0	1	2
I judge myself by what I accomplish, not by how busy I am.	0	1	2
I (and not *circumstances* or *other people's* priorities) control my own daily schedule and activities.	0	1	2
I have a clear idea of what I want to accomplish during the coming months.	0	1	2
I'm satisfied with the way I use my time.	0	1	2
Total score (the sum of all your item scores)	0	1	2

Look at your total score. If it's between 35 and 40, you're probably pretty organized and you likely manage your time wisely. If you scored between 30 and 34, you're probably staying afloat, but your time management skills could use a tune-up. If your score was below 30, read this chapter carefully and use all the worksheets. Among the time management skills you'll learn are how to organize your priorities, avoid becoming overcommitted, and gain more control over your time. Unfortunately, unless you learn these skills and take steps to begin to effectively solve personal time management problems, your life is likely to remain stressful and less than satisfying.

MATTERS OF IMPORTANCE VERSUS MATTERS OF URGENCY: HOW DO YOU SPEND YOUR TIME?

Stress increases when you spend your time in ways that don't help you achieve what you want out of life. The more your day-to-day, hour-to-hour, moment-to-moment activities are out of sync with your goals and ideals, the more you get stressed. Alden loved managing his resort hotel and wanted it to be successful so that he could enjoy a comfortable and fulfilling family life. But he became a victim of circumstances. When the work piled up, even after hiring extra staff, Alden took on extra tasks that he could have shared or delegated. He began responding too much to matters of *urgency* (relatively minor problems that crop up here and there) rather than to matters of *importance*—the things that align most closely with his life's ambitions. As a result, Alden felt unfulfilled and stressed.

What Are Your Life's Ambitions?

Like Alden, we all deal with both urgent and important matters in our daily lives. When you give priority to the *important* matters, you spend more time planning and preparing to meet valuable goals that satisfy your ambitions. You have more control over how you're spending your time, and this makes you feel productive—like you're spending your time wisely. If you let the *urgent* matters win the day, you end up with more stress because more of your time is controlled by external factors over which you have less control. You spend your time putting out little fires and responding to other people's requests, which are less meaningful to you.

What are the things in life that are most important to you? How can you spend more of your time on these people, tasks, and activities and less time responding to circumstances? These are crucial issues to resolve when learning how to manage your time.

Of course, not all matters of urgency are unimportant; sometimes they're critical (for example, responding to an emergency or acting on a boss's orders). In fact, most matters involve some degree of both importance *and* urgency. But before you can decide how to allocate your time among the important, the urgent, and the important-and-urgent, you need to identify the things in your life that are truly important to you. Who are the people that matter most to you (at home, work, school, or otherwise)? Which relationships are worth investing your valuable time in? What are you passionate about? What energizes and inspires you to leap out of bed in the morning? What would you like to learn more about? What would you like to do better? Are you comfortable financially? Do you need to increase your earning potential? What problems do you need to solve in your life? Everyone has unique goals and values. Consider the questions in this paragraph and, in the spaces below, write down at least ten things in life that are very important to you—your passions, goals, values. Alden's list was as follows:

1. Relationship with my wife

2. Relationship with my children

3. Financial stability

4. Reducing my stress level

5. Managing my hotel

6. Friends

7. Baseball (my favorite team and my fantasy baseball team)

8. Playing the guitar (becoming a better player)

9. Interest in American history

10. Traveling the world

What are *your* matters of importance?

1. _____

2. _____

3. _____

4. _____

5. _____

6. _____

7. _____

8. _____

9. _____

10. _____

Where Does Your Time Go?

Now, how much time do you actually spend on these matters versus matters of urgency? And how much time is simply wasted? Chances are that, knowing this, you'll be able to reduce some stress by setting new priorities and increasing your time spent on the important matters. Most of us underestimate how long we spend doing various tasks, and we tend to forget about unplanned activities that crop up through the day. So, simply *thinking about* or trying to remember where your time goes isn't going to work very well. Instead, you'll need to use a diary or journal, such as the Activity Log on page 133, to keep track of your daily activities for at least 3 days. (If this seems like it will just take up more of your valuable time, remember that the time you invest now will save you much more time later.) Here are some suggestions for filling out the Activity Log.

- Fill it out in "real time" throughout the day, rather than waiting until the end of the day, when you're tired and likely to forget or underestimate important things. This means you'll need to take the log with you and have it handy throughout the day. Make sure you record *everything* you spend more than a few minutes doing.

- In the far left column, note the time of day when you started and finished the activity. Try to be exact—use a clock or watch.

- There's no need to be overly detailed; just use terms that will allow you to recognize the activity upon reviewing the log: e-mailing, meeting, answering phone calls, socializing, eating, conference call, child care, shopping, daydreaming, surfing the Web, cooking, driving, watching TV, playing ball, napping, and so on.

- Rate your level of stress over the task from 0 (none) to 4 (intense).

- If you have any comments about doing the activity, enter them in the "Remarks" column.

- Don't do anything with the "Category" column. We'll get to this later.

- Make copies of the blank form for future use and log your activities for at least 3 "typical" days.

- Use Alden's sample Activity Log on page 134 as an example.

Learning from Your Activity Log

Now that we have some data about how you're spending your time, let's analyze it and find out how much your daily activities match up with your goals and values. Do you need to adjust the amount of time you spend each day on the important matters in your life? To find out, follow these steps:

- First, review your logs to see if you can pick out any patterns in your behavior. Are you especially productive or unproductive at certain times of the day? Are certain activities particularly stressful? What did you learn about how you spend your time?

_____

_____

- Second, identify the activities that are in line with the things you listed on page 131 as important matters in your life. In the far right column (labeled "Category") of the Activity Log, circle _I_ if an activity is related to one of these important matters.

Glance at Alden's forms. He circled _I_'s for activities that involved spending time with his family, being productive at work, and spending time reading about baseball—which he followed closely (see Alden's important matters on page 130).

- Third, identify activities that you did because they were urgent instead of important—that you did because external pressure made you feel like you had to get something done. In the "Category" column of the Activity Log, circle _U_ for each of these activities.

Alden's urgent activities involved putting out fires that could have been handled by other people, but that Alden felt he _had_ to deal with to make sure they were done just right. In addition to changing lightbulbs, these included spending too much time training new employees, trying to fix computer glitches, and changing his plans to meet with the hotel landscaper who showed up on the wrong day for an appointment. Alden could have delegated most of these tasks to others, thereby increasing his time available for more crucial and important matters. Once he realized how much time he was spending putting out fires and doing things that could be delegated, he made up his mind to assign more responsibilities to the people he managed at the hotel.

ACTIVITY LOG (DATE: _____)

Time	Activity	Stress rating	Remarks	Category
		0 1 2 3 4		I U W
		0 1 2 3 4		I U W
		0 1 2 3 4		I U W
		0 1 2 3 4		I U W
		0 1 2 3 4		I U W
		0 1 2 3 4		I U W
		0 1 2 3 4		I U W
		0 1 2 3 4		I U W
		0 1 2 3 4		I U W
		0 1 2 3 4		I U W
		0 1 2 3 4		I U W
		0 1 2 3 4		I U W
		0 1 2 3 4		I U W
		0 1 2 3 4		I U W
		0 1 2 3 4		I U W
		0 1 2 3 4		I U W
		0 1 2 3 4		I U W
		0 1 2 3 4		I U W
		0 1 2 3 4		I U W

Stress rating: 0 = No stress, 1 = Low, 2 = Moderate, 3 = High, 4 = Extreme

ACTIVITY LOG: ALDEN (DATE: _MONDAY, JUNE 23_)

Time	Activity	Stress rating	Remarks	Category
6:15–6:50	Wake up, shower, get dressed, wake up kids	0 1 ②3 4	Woke up stressed out just thinking about the day.	①U W
6:50–7:30	Breakfast with kids	0①2 3 4		①U W
7:30–7:45	Take Noah to bus	⓪1 2 3 4		①U W
7:45–8:20	Drive to work	0 1 2③4	Traffic not as bad as usual	①U W
8:20–8:50	Online—read and answer e-mail, read about last night's baseball games, web surfing	0 1②3 4	Back and forth between actual work and reading sports websites	①U Ⓦ
9:00–10:00	Staff meeting	0 1②3 4	Introduced Jocelyn—new staff member	①U W
10:00–10:45	Answer e-mails, return calls	0 1 2③4	Lots to return	①U W
10:45–11:30	Train Jocelyn on desk duty	0 1 2 3④	Mark or Ron could do this	I Ⓤ W
11:30–11:45	Change light bulbs in lobby	0 1 2 3④		I Ⓤ W
11:45–1:00	Office: paperwork, phone calls	0 1 2③4		①U W
1:00–2:30	Out to lunch with Mark & Ron, call Sandra [wife]	0①2 3 4	Waited in line at Remy's for 30 minutes!	①U Ⓦ
2:30–3:30	Visit with Mark in his office	0 1②3 4	We mainly talked about sports	I U Ⓦ
3:30–4:40	Meet with new landscaper and give a tour	0 1②3 4	Showed up on the wrong day. I had planned to do other work.	I Ⓤ W
4:40–5:00	Tried to fix a computer issue	0 1 2 3④	Ended up calling IT anyway	I Ⓤ W
5:10–6:10	Help at front desk, check up on valet	0 1 2 3④	Spent too much time doing this	①U W
6:10–6:30	Facebook, surfing the web for things to buy on eBay, read news online	0 1 2③4	We don't really need a new website	I U Ⓦ
6:30–7:00	Drive home	0 1 2 3④	Traffic!	①U W
7:20–7:45	Dinner with Sandra	0①2 3 4		①U W
7:45–8:15	Play/read with Noah and Olivia	⓪1 2 3 4		①U W
8:15–8:30	Tuck kids in bed	⓪1 2 3 4		①U W
8:30–8:50	Answer e-mails, check voice mail	0 1 2③4		I Ⓤ W
8:50–9:25	Talk with Sandra while watching TV	0①2 3 4		①U W
9:30–10:00	Snack/TV with Sandra	0①2 3 4		①U W

You can do the same thing. Look over the activities you marked *U* and consider how you could reduce or eliminate them from your daily schedule. Write down some ideas for doing so:

_____

_____

- Finally, for any activity that represents a waste of time—that is, it doesn't accomplish anything important or urgent—circle *W* in the far right column of the Activity Log.

Alden found that he occasionally spent too much time at the computer just surfing the Web or looking for things to buy. His lunch break, which he found only *somewhat* productive and important (he checked in with his wife and discussed some work matters with his coworkers), also took too much time (notice that an activity can be both important and a waste of time if, for example, it takes too long). Finally, he noticed that he had a tendency to visit and chat with coworkers about non-work-related matters. Alden decided he would try limiting his lunch break to a maximum of 30 minutes and begin bringing a packed lunch from home to cut down on time (and calories).

Everyone wastes some of their time each day doing things that are neither productive nor urgent. That's generally okay, although people who manage their time well are able to minimize how much time they spend this way so it doesn't interfere with productivity. Examine your sources of wasted time and think about what you could do to reduce or eliminate them. What ideas can you come up with?

_____

_____

_____

Now take what you've learned about yourself and the ideas you've come up with in this section to improve how you manage your time. Increasing your time spent doing activities related to important goals and values will help reduce your stress and make you more productive. Go slowly—don't try to make too many changes at once or you risk feeling overwhelmed and scrapping your plans altogether. Instead, alter your routine a bit at a time—adding one new change each week. Over time, the changes will add up and you'll find yourself being more productive and satisfied. On the Weekly Changes worksheet on the next page, arrange your ideas for reducing urgent and wasteful activities in an action plan. Specify which idea you'll try out each week for the next several weeks. This will help you keep track of your plan to make gradual changes in your time management.

Time is a valuable resource. When you invest it wisely in the here and now, it yields important long-term returns.

WEEKLY CHANGES

Week of (date)   Changes I will make this week:

_____   _____

_____   _____

_____   _____

_____   _____

_____   _____

_____   _____

_____   _____

EYE 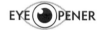 PENER

Counting *I*'s and *U*'s

Count the number of *I*'s and *U*'s that you circled on your Activity Logs. If your urgent activities outnumber the important ones, something's wrong. Spending too much time on urgent matters takes time away from those that are most fulfilling. Maybe you put less time into your relationships or deny yourself much needed relaxation and leisure time. You might even forgo physical exercise and healthy eating habits—which are also very important. When you neglect these and other important activities, your days will seem long, exhausting, and stressful. Improving your time management skills will help you break this pattern.

GETTING ORGANIZED

Now that you're aware of the kinds of changes that could help you improve your time management, let's move on to some specific ways to stay organized and save time. Many of the tools and techniques in this section will be familiar. You may have tried some of them without much improvement, so I've concentrated on offering tips for maximizing the effectiveness of these tools. Feeling disorganized is a major stressor for many people because it makes you feel scattered and unfocused on top of not getting enough done.

Get the Most Out of Your Planner or Calendar

Keeping track of your daily, weekly, and monthly commitments, whether with a paper calendar, a PDA, or a smartphone, is critical to staying organized, even if you think you have the best memory in the world. But there are ways to make it work as well as it should:

- Remember that *what doesn't get scheduled doesn't get done.* So enter each task hanging over your head whether you're absolutely sure you can get it done when scheduled or not. It will have a much better chance of getting done if it's on your agenda.

- Make sure you have only one planner. Having different tasks and events in different planners is almost as ineffective as having no planner at all.

- Make sure the size and shape allow you to take your planner with you wherever you go.

- Be sure the format and layout work for you. If there's not enough room for the detail you need, you'll opt out of entering important events and tasks.

- If it's electronic, is it easy to use on the go?

- Put *everything* in your planner: meetings, appointments, class times, presentations, deadlines and due dates, exams, birthdays, and so on—your organizer is "information central."

Keep a To-Do List Simple to Make It Work

A to-do list should serve as an at-a-glance reminder if it's to do its job:

- When something to do comes up, just add it to your list, whether on a paper pad or electronically. Don't waste time trying to list things in order of priority. If your eye can run down the list easily, you'll prioritize just by glancing at your list periodically.

- Have only one to-do list. As with planners, if your entries aren't all in one place, the list loses its utility.

- Don't waste time managing your list or worrying about how neat it looks. Simply write down what you need to do.

- Cross off tasks as soon as you've completed them—it's the most satisfying part of all and will give you incentive to keep tackling the rest of the list.

Delegate Thoughtfully

If you're at all like Alden, chances are you feel you're the best person to get the job—any job that matters to you—done. But you might be surprised at how much others are motivated or how easily they can be taught. And even if other people can't do the job as

EYE PENER

Reducing Low-Priority Activities

Be selective in how you choose to spend your time. Find ways to remove activities from your schedule that are less important or that take too much time away from working toward your goals. Do you go to every social occasion (parties, dinners, gatherings) that you're invited to? These can take up lots of time, but you don't have to attend them all. It's the same for meetings—the PTA, congregational meetings, neighborhood or tenant meetings, and other organizations you might belong to. Attend these if you really want or need to; but if not, give yourself permission to put the time to use in other (more productive) ways. Be assertive— people won't dislike you because you have other things to do with your time; for example, "Thank you for your invitation, but I've got so much on my plate right now that I have to decline. Thanks for understanding."

well as you can, you're *still* better off delegating some of the work than taking it all on yourself and feeling extremely stressed. Here are some suggestions for delegating successfully at work and at home:

- Delegate responsibilities only to people you have confidence in. Make sure they have the know-how to get the job done. If no one else seems to fit the bill, consider investing the time to train someone.

- Boost other people's interest in working hard for you by offering praise and letting them know why you've chosen them for the job. Show them how much you appreciate the time they're giving up to help you out. You might say something like "I've noticed that you're terrific at graphic design. I realize you're very busy, but I'd be grateful if you'd please help put together the PowerPoint slides for the presentation." (Notice the assertive tone and the *I* statement; see Chapter 6 for details on these skills.)

- Don't hover—no one likes to be micromanaged. So, once you've delegated *and clearly explained* what you want the other person to do, stand back and let him or her do it. Step in and offer assistance only if asked or if you should somehow learn that there's been a total meltdown.

- Be assertive. When you delegate tasks to others—colleagues at work, friends, or family members—do so with self-confidence and don't feel guilty. Use *I* statements and appropriate body language. If you're wishy-washy in your request, the other person won't take you as seriously.

Now let's figure out what you could delegate to whom. Carefully consider what you just read about delegating. Then think about jobs and tasks at home, work, and so on that you could give to others to allow you more time for truly important matters. Write these down in the worksheet below.

Don't Waste Time Making Minor Decisions

Do you ever find yourself having to make choices between similarly appealing, or relatively unimportant, options? Elana was trying to decide whether to use pink or yellow icing to decorate her daughter's birthday cake. Ron saw two shirts he really liked but couldn't choose one to buy. Save time and avoid agonizing over these sorts of decisions:

- Flip a coin if you can't decide quickly.

- Ask yourself whether your decision matters more than the time you'll save.

DELEGATING TASKS

Tasks I can delegate	Person (people) I can delegate to
1.	
2.	
3.	
4.	
5.	
6.	
7.	

Multitask the Right Way

Multitasking can help you get things done—as long as you make the right choices of tasks to do simultaneously:

- Choose mainly habitual and routine tasks to do at the same time: reading your favorite news website or listening to the news and weather while you eat breakfast or put on your makeup; watching your favorite show (or the big game) while you fold laundry, cook, or assemble that new bookshelf you bought for your living room; writing letters or studying while you're waiting at the doctor's office or riding the bus.

- Don't talk on the phone, read, send e-mails or text messages, or eat while you're driving. Anything that requires your full attention for safety's sake should be done by itself.

- Don't try to multitask when you're trying to learn new tasks, focusing on a complex task, or doing activities involving planning. The parts of the brain that help you do these kinds of activities require your undivided attention.

Think about ways you can multitask your own activities. Write them in the following spaces:

_____

_____

_____

_____

- Bundle similar tasks together. For instance, rather than interrupting your schedule to answer and return each e-mail or phone call you get, wait until several have piled up and then return them all in one session. It's the same with paying bills. Plan a time each month when you'll pay all of the bills that have accumulated since last month. What tasks can you bundle together? Write these down in the following spaces:

_____

_____

_____

_____

Use Spare Time Wisely

A little extra time can be a gift, but don't squander it:

- Don't try to squeeze in large or important tasks. You'll only put pressure on yourself and end up disappointed with how much you *don't* get done.

- Use small amounts of spare time to catch up on simpler things such as making phone calls, chatting with a friend, or writing e-mails or letters.

- Use waiting time between meetings or classes to be productive too. Check over an assignment that needs to be turned in or review your class notes. You could even use the time to catch up on reading about your favorite sport or hobby.

What can you do when you have spare or extra time? Write these down in the following spaces:

_____

_____

_____

_____

Take Breaks That Increase Productivity

You may think the last thing you have time for is time off, but taking breaks will make your active time more productive:

- Even a break as short as 5 minutes will help.

- Make breaks frequent—every hour or so.

- Get a change of scenery, clear your head, take in some fresh air, and most of all, get your blood pumping again. Taking a walk through the building, or even around the block outside, is the perfect break.

Match Your Activities with Your Energy Levels

Sometimes you have all the energy in the world. You're *in the zone* and feel like you could eat an elephant all at once! But let's face it, sometimes you just don't feel like working. Whether it's because your attitude is off or your energy level is low, you just don't feel like doing anything. People who are good at managing their time, though, know how to sort their tasks by energy (or motivational) level so that they stay productive no matter how they feel. And so can you:

- When your energy level is high and you're at your most alert (in the morning for many people), tackle big, important tasks that require lots of concentration and persistence, such as yardwork, creative work, writing, studying, brainstorming and strategy sessions, and holding meetings with other people (clients, colleagues, professors, study groups).

- When your energy level is lower and you feel like calling it a day, take on low-effort tasks that don't require much concentration or follow-through, including making phone calls, writing letters and e-mails, cleaning up, organizing your space and filing papers, and working out (that's right—this can actually make you perk up).

- Learn to recognize your energy level patterns through the day. Use the worksheet below to help you.

SCHEDULING TASKS ACCORDING TO ENERGY LEVEL

My high-energy times of the day: _____

Activities for these times: _____

_____

_____

_____

My low-energy times of the day: _____

Activities for these times: _____

_____

_____

_____

Play Hard to Work Hard

Your *work–life balance* refers to how you prioritize between your career and other ambitions on the one hand and pleasure, leisure, health, and family matters on the other. As people who are good at time management are aware, it's important to schedule opportunities to relax, have fun, and take part in enjoyable activities. Here are some ideas for scheduling play so that you have something to look forward to; a break from your daily routine that will make you feel refreshed when you get back to work:

- Schedule leisure for just an hour or two a few times a week. If you try to take a whole day off, you might feel so guilty that it will only cause you more stress.

- Choose something that *you* find relaxing and rejuvenating—whether it's a visit to the spa or fitness club, a "day date" or romantic encounter with someone special, a manicure/pedicure, or lunch with friends—not something that conventional wisdom or other people designate as leisure activities but that you don't enjoy.

- Give these activities a specific slot in your schedule using your planner; otherwise you may decide you don't have time for them and keep putting them off. Using your planner can also ensure that your leisure activities don't interfere with your productivity. If you don't schedule diversions, you may be prone to blow off something important to run out and play just because you can't stand to work one more second. In the following spaces, write down leisure activities you'd like to schedule into your routine. Then go to your planner and look for ways you can fit them in.

_____

_____

_____

PROCRASTINATION

At last, here's the section on procrastination! We procrastinate when we put off important, high-priority (often unpleasant) tasks until "later" and instead engage in less important (often more enjoyable) activities in the here and now. Everyone does it, and a certain amount of procrastination is perfectly normal. But if it's excessive, or you procrastinate on tasks that are too important to leave undone, it's a habit that can result in a lot of stress. Maybe you avoid tasks you dislike but then can't put them off any longer and pull all-nighters to meet deadlines. Or you wait so long that your performance at work or school slumps. Or you suffer social disapproval for not meeting your commitments. Any of these consequences of procrastination can produce even more stress than you might have suffered just from doing what you didn't want to do.

> *Lost time is never found.*

How much of a problem is procrastination for you? Rate the statements in the form on the facing page based on how true they are of you by circling a number from 1 (not at all true of me) to 5 (very true of me).

Once you've filled out the worksheet, add up your scores and write the total down here: _____. A lower number is better. If your total score was between 10 and 20, you tend not to allow your to-do list to get too long and instead take action as soon as possible. You probably procrastinate very little and won't need the tips in this section. If you scored between 21 and 30, procrastination might be a factor in some of your problems with time management . . . and stress. Although it might not be a serious burden, it's a problem worth solving. Finally, if you scored between 31 and 50, you're probably procrastinating more than is good for you, and your time management difficulties are likely causing you stress. In this section, I'll give you some tried-and-true strategies for turning things around. Read on—don't put this off!

Analyzing Your Procrastination

Really digging in and trying to understand a problem puts you in the best position to solve it. Procrastination can be a way of coping with stress over starting or completing a task—a very challenging work project, studying for an exam, and calling someone to offer condolences for the loss of their loved one might be examples. It might be in response to having to make a difficult or uncomfortable decision, such as which house or car to buy. You might procrastinate because you're concerned you don't have the skills to do a good job. Other times people procrastinate simply to put off tedious tasks, such as house or yard work. Regardless, behind procrastination are usually thoughts and beliefs such as "I'll be in a better mood to do this later," "I'm good at getting things done at the last minute," and "I'll put this off until I know how to do it perfectly." You might sometimes feel that you don't deserve to have to work or be stressed out; for example, "I shouldn't ruin the day by doing things I don't want to do." Take a look at the Procrastination Analysis worksheet on the facing page and see if you can identify why you're putting off certain obligations.

It's best to complete this form when you're in the midst of procrastinating—like when you've got that gnawing feeling that you *should* get to work on an unpleasant task or job, but you find yourself looking for reasons not to. In the first column of the worksheet, describe the task you're putting off. Then list the reasons you're putting it off. These might be many or few. Seth, who has procrastination problems, also completed the worksheet. Take a look at his example on page 147 to help you complete your form.

The next step is to confront and challenge the reasons for putting off the activity. Indeed, some things in life are unpleasant, and we can all think of many things we'd rather be doing instead. But at the same time, there are positive reasons for moving ahead and just getting these tasks over with. There might be tangible benefits to getting the job

IS PROCRASTINATION STRESSING YOU OUT?

1. I leave projects until the last minute.	1 2 3 4 5
2. I pull all-nighters to get things done on time.	1 2 3 4 5
3. When I'm stressed, I watch TV, chat, or surf the Web instead of working.	1 2 3 4 5
4. I can usually find reasons for putting off unpleasant activities until later.	1 2 3 4 5
5. I'm late with paying bills (even when I have enough money in my account).	1 2 3 4 5
6. I miss deadlines.	1 2 3 4 5
7. There are things I should do that I've been putting off for weeks or months.	1 2 3 4 5
8. I have to find the "right time" to do certain things.	1 2 3 4 5
9. It can take me several days to respond to e-mail or voicemail messages.	1 2 3 4 5
10. I put off doing things around the house for days, such as the dishes, laundry, taking out the trash, and other sorts of routine task and chores.	1 2 3 4 5

PROCRASTINATION ANALYSIS

Task I'm putting off	Why I'm putting off doing this task	Confronting my reasons for putting it off	My new plan

done (for example, the house will smell fresher once it's cleaned), feelings of accomplishment (pride that you did something important today), or just relief that the unpleasant task is out of the way ("Yes! At last, *that's* over with"). Check out what Seth wrote and then, for each reason to put your task off, come up with at least one positive reason for going ahead with it.

Finally, set some goals and develop a plan for completing the task immediately. Maybe you'll break it down into steps. Maybe you'll reward yourself for getting it done more quickly—like Seth decided to do. Write your plan in the last column of the worksheet and then get started!

More Tips for Reducing Procrastination

When you really analyze your reasons for putting off a task, and then challenge the thoughts and beliefs behind your procrastination, you're likely to see that you can come up with alternative ways to think about the situation or task that lead to getting it done sooner rather than later. But overcoming procrastination requires having a number of tricks up your sleeve. Here are some additional ideas to use the next time you're tempted to put off something you don't want to do.

Pros and Cons

Make two lists: the first is a list of all the unpleasant aspects of doing the task that you're currently putting off. In the second list, write down the consequences of putting off the task. On the facing page you can see the lists that Larry, a teacher, made about getting started with grading a stack of his students' papers, which he'd been putting off.

These lists in hand, Larry then carefully contemplated the discomfort of grading his class's papers versus the consequences of putting this off even further—you should do this with your lists as well—and realized that the consequences of *not* grading the papers would actually be *more* unpleasant than just grading them here and now. It was the lesser of two evils. And thinking about it this way motivated him to set aside the time and grade the papers right away. Try this exercise the next time you're procrastinating. You'll probably arrive at the same conclusions and (hopefully) make the same decision.

Link the Unpleasant Task to a Pleasant One

Like the spoonful of sugar that helps the medicine go down, when you connect an activity you don't enjoy (the "medicine") with something you like (the "sugar"), suddenly the unlikable activity doesn't seem so bad. If, for example, you're putting off unloading the dishwasher or doing other work around the house, try linking it to something you like such as putting on your favorite music and "rocking out" while you clean or work. If you dislike exercising or grocery shopping, get a friend to go with you who can chat with you, show you some new exercise moves, or help you find bargains.

PROCRASTINATION ANALYSIS: SETH

Task I'm putting off	Why I'm putting off doing this task	Confronting my reasons for putting it off	My new plan
Mowing the lawn	• It takes up 45 minutes. • It's boring. • I don't <u>have</u> to do it today. It could wait until another day.	• 45 minutes is a short time in the scheme of things. • I can listen to music on my iPod to make it more interesting. • I don't have to do it today, but I'll sure feel better when it's done.	Go take 45 minutes to mow the lawn while listening to music; and then relax with a snack while watching the game.

PROS AND CONS OF DOING A TASK: LARRY

Unpleasant aspects of grading papers	Consequences of not grading the papers
• It will take a long time. • It's monotonous. • There are so many other, more interesting things I could be doing.	• I'll still have to do it at some point—the papers won't grade themselves. • There will be even more papers to grade soon, so my work will only pile up and make me more stressed. • My students will be upset because I have been delaying getting their papers back to them and they want to know how they did on the assignments. • If a student isn't doing well, I won't know and can't help them.

Reward Yourself

When all else fails, set up a reward system in which you earn points for completing the tasks you've been putting off. Make a list, and when you've earned a certain number of points, buy yourself something special.

Break the Task into Pieces

This is pretty self-explanatory. If the whole task or job seems overwhelming and difficult to tackle all at once, there's no harm in breaking it down into smaller and more manageable ("bite-sized") tasks that you can feel better about doing.

So, now that you've got a better understanding of how you spend your time, and some strategies to improve your time management, you can begin making changes to reduce your stress. But go gradually. If you try to change too much too fast, you risk not being able to keep up with all of your adjustments, which can lead to feeling overwhelmed—exactly what you're trying to avoid. I recommend trying out one new time management strategy per week. Once you're comfortable with using this new strategy, try adding another each week until you feel you're making progress.

8

Changing Your Stressful Thinking

As you learned in Chapter 3, stress and other emotional responses are not caused by situations and events, but rather by thoughts, beliefs, interpretations, and assumptions (*cognitions*) *about* situations and events. Negative emotions come from your interpretations, and when those interpretations are faulty—exaggerated, inaccurate, and otherwise unhelpful—they can lead to excessive stress. That's called the *cognitive principle*, and *cognitive-behavioral therapy* (CBT) is the basis for the strategies you'll learn in this chapter for correcting problematic thoughts to reduce stress.

To understand how the cognitive principle works, consider how Laura might react if she took a world history exam on Friday and then her professor approached her on Monday and said, "Laura, see me after class today." What emotion do you think Laura would be experiencing as she sat there in class waiting to meet with her professor? How would she feel?

> *Remember the cognitive principle: It's not so much what's happening to you that determines your stress level. It's how you interpret what's happening.*

It all depends on her interpretation—*what she tells herself about the situation she's in.* Here are some possibilities:

- "Uh-oh; I probably failed the exam and Dr. Jenkins is very angry. What's he going to do to me?" → **Anxiety**

- "Dr. Jenkins is an idiot! He shouldn't make me wait through class to talk to him!" → **Anger**

- "I probably failed the exam. I can't do anything right. I'm a loser." → **Sadness**

- "Oh, good. Now I'll have a chance to explain my answers on the exam." → **Relief**

- "Dr. Jenkins wants to get to know me a little better." → **Calmness**

What Laura told herself about the situation created her reality and dictated how she felt. This relationship applies to most situations in life. When you feel *anxious*, it's because your thoughts are focused on themes of threat, danger, or unpredictability. *Anger* occurs when you think about others behaving in ways you don't like (as if they're deliberately violating your rules). Feelings of *sadness* or *depression* result when your thoughts concern loss, hopelessness, or helplessness. Positive feelings of *relief* occur when you tell yourself that a potential threat has been lifted. And feelings of *calmness* are the result of neutral or pleasant thoughts.

THE COGNITIVE PRINCIPLE AND STRESS

Exaggerated and self-defeating cognitions are the foundation of problems with stress. Shawn was stressed out over his recent problems with sexual functioning and had worked himself up into believing that he was "less of a man" because he couldn't maintain erections long enough for satisfying intercourse with his wife. He believed it was just a matter of time before his wife decided to leave him for a "real man." From the cognitive perspective, Shawn's beliefs (for example, "My wife will leave me because of my sexual problem") led him to feel extremely stressed and anxious (which only put more strain on their marriage and made Shawn's erectile dysfunction difficulties worse).

But are sexual problems in men really a sign of weakness, as Shawn believed? Was his wife really about to leave him over this? Shawn never made any effort to check out whether his beliefs were correct. He just *assumed* they were because of comments and jokes he'd heard from other men. And he never bothered to discuss his concerns with his wife to find out how she felt. So Shawn went on believing that his assumptions were correct—which kept him very stressed.

Had Shawn taken the time to look into whether his cognitions were accurate, he would have discovered that most men experience sexual performance difficulties from time to time and that this problem is highly treatable. And he would have found out that his wife had never even considered leaving. Had he known all of this, Shawn would have changed his self-defeating cognitions into more realistic beliefs, such as "This is a real nuisance, but I can get help; and it's not a threat to my marriage." These beliefs would have reduced Shawn's stress level and maybe even helped boost his sexual performance without requiring professional help.

Stressful thinking patterns escalate your stress. If you reduce stressful thinking, you'll reduce your stress level.

Shawn could have used problem solving (Chapter 5) to figure out that his erectile dysfunction could be treated effectively. But modifying the problem situation would take time, and meanwhile he might still be under a lot of stress worrying about whether treatment would be successful, whether his sex life would be permanently altered, and whether his wife was going to leave him. The beauty of the cognitive approach is that it can help you reduce stress even when you cannot control the problem at hand by using problem solving, assertiveness (Chapter 6), or time management (Chapter 7). With cognitive strategies, come what may, you'll be in control of your emotions. You won't have to depend on everything (and *everyone*) being just right for you to feel less stressed. Here's another example:

Maria received a phone call—her mother had felt a very small lump on her breast but couldn't see the doctor until a few days later. Maria panicked: "Oh my God, Mom's going to die of breast cancer!" she told herself. "What will I do without her!?" When her stress level intensified, Maria turned to cognitive therapy. She recognized that her thinking processes were exaggerated: Not yet knowing her mother's diagnosis, she was jumping to conclusions. So she challenged herself to change her thinking. For instance, she hadn't considered that her mother had caught the lump early and that it might be benign. And although it's nothing to take lightly, many more women survive breast cancer today than in years past. Considering these facts helped weaken Maria's exaggerated cognitions to the point that she could feel appropriately *concerned* rather than extremely stressed and panicked.

Accurate, not *Positive*, Thinking

If you're highly stressed, there are probably more accurate ways of thinking about the things that are happening to (or around) you. But *accurate* thinking is not the same as *positive* thinking. And you shouldn't confuse cognitive therapy, which is about thinking accurately and logically, with simply trying to replace negative thoughts with positive ones. The so-called "power of positive thinking" might be helpful for some difficulties, but it's not a good strategy for combating stress. You'll get much better results with logical thinking. Why? Because logical thoughts can be verified, they're believable, and they're not rigid or absolutistic.

And let's face it, there are times in life when it's perfectly appropriate to feel annoyed, sad, or concerned. So, trying to be happy and positive all the time—especially if you lead a high-stress life—is not practical. The comparison below shows how cognitive therapy aims to transform your intense, unhelpful (and highly stressful) negative emotions into feelings and emotions that are more moderate, adaptive, less stressful, and easier to manage.

Intense, irrational, and maladaptive stress-provoking emotion	Moderate, adaptive, logical, and stress-reducing emotion
Anger, rage, frustration	Annoyed, displeased, irked
Depressed, miserable, guilty	Sad, upset, disappointed
Anxious, fearful, worried	Concerned, uneasy

BACK TO ABC

In Chapter 3 (page 44) I introduced the cognitive model of emotion using the ABC framework in which A is the stressful event that *activates* the emotional response, B is the thinking pattern or *belief system* that intensifies negative emotions about A, and C represents the emotional and behavioral *consequences* of the thoughts and beliefs. You also learned about six thinking patterns that lead to stress. If it's been a while since you reviewed this material, you might as well read through pages 50–56 again to refresh your memory. Before you can use cognitive therapy strategies to modify stress-related thinking, you need to figure out which faulty thinking patterns cause you the greatest stress. That's the point of the ABC Log on the facing page. Before going further in this chapter, spend a few days to a week using the log to keep track of how your thinking patterns influence your stress. This will help you get familiar with the particular cognitions that you'll want to modify using the cognitive therapy strategies.

Here's how to use the log (a few examples appear on page 154):

1. Keep copies of the form with you throughout the day to fill out when you're feeling stressed. Make several copies so you don't run out.

2. When you notice your stress level rising, note the date and time and put a brief description of the A—the activating event that triggered the stress—in the first column of the form. For example, "Joanne didn't invite me for the holidays" or "We lost a lot of money in the stock market this quarter."

3. Then, in the second column, write down your B's—the stressful beliefs and assumptions about the situation at A. We sometimes call these cognitions *automatic thoughts* since they can occur without your even being aware. That means you might need to think carefully about what's going through your mind. The best way to do that is to ask yourself questions such as the following:

   - "What am I telling myself about the stressful event?"
   - "What is the worst thing about this situation?"
   - "What am I afraid might happen?"
   - "What does this say about me, my life, my future?"
   - "What might other people be thinking about me?"
   - "What does this say about the other person (or people—or the world—in general)?"

   Finally, keep in mind that for any A you might have only one, or multiple B's. When you notice more than one, write them all down. For example, "Joanne didn't invite me because she thinks I'm no fun" and "I'm such a failure for losing money in the stock market."

4. In the column marked "Type of stress-related thinking pattern," label each B according to the types of stress-related cognitions. Again, reread pages 50–56

ABC LOG

A *Activating* event (and date/time)	B *Beliefs* and other cognitions about "A"	Type of stress- related thinking patterns	C *Consequences* (strength of your emotional response)

ABC LOG: EXAMPLES

A *Activating* event (and date/time)	B *Beliefs* and other cognitions about "A"	Type of stress- related thinking patterns	C *Consequences* (strength of your emotional response)
March 23 Waiting in line at the bank	"I can't stand being late!" "They should have more tellers available to help out." "I'll walk in late to the meeting and everyone will think I'm disorganized."	• I-can't-stand-its • <u>Must</u>urbation • Jumping to conclusions	• Stressed 7 • Angry 8
September 18 Someone broke into my car and stole my wallet, among other things	"I'm a loser for leaving my wallet in the car." "I always get the bad luck." "This is horrible! I'll never get back what was taken."	• Labeling • All-or-nothing thinking • Awfulizing • Jumping to conclusions	Depressed 7 Stressed 9 Anxious 6

if you need a review of how to identify each thinking pattern. Here's a list of them:

- All-or-nothing (black-and-white) thinking
- *Must*urbation
- Jumping to conclusions
- Awfulizing
- "I-can't-stand-its"
- Labeling

5. Finally, in the last column, note your emotional response (emotions and feelings are usually recorded with one-word descriptions such as *anxiety, stress, depression, anger*, and so on) and its intensity on a scale from 0 (very weak) to 10 (extremely intense). I recommend using the log anytime an A activates a stress level of at least 5.

After you've spent some time keeping track of your thinking habits in different stressful situations, look for patterns. Do you notice certain stress-related thinking patterns that come up time and time again? In the following space, write down the three patterns you found that you used most often:

1. _____

2. _____

3. _____

These thinking patterns will be your *main* targets when you begin using the cognitive therapy techniques described next. That's not to say your other thinking patterns aren't important, just that you need to start somewhere.

CHANGING STRESSFUL THINKING PATTERNS

All-or-Nothing (Black-and-White) Thinking

Thinking in absolutes—seeing things as either totally *perfect* or utterly *horrible*—oversimplifies real life and amplifies the negative. The real world isn't black and white. In fact, absolute perfection is more or less an illusion—as is absolute *disaster*. But when you see things in black and white, anything short of perfection seems like a disaster. Getting a score of 90% on an exam, for example, feels the same as getting an F. What an unfortunate way to live! Here are some strategies for challenging and moving beyond all-or-nothing thinking. Do you find yourself thinking this way?

Seeing the Shades of Gray

If you think about it, there are "degrees of badness" in even the most stressful experiences life throws at you. And recognizing the "shades of gray" is the best antidote to all-or-nothing thinking. Take Derrick, a teacher who was forced to take a salary cut because of changes to the school system's budget. He said that his life was "a complete disaster," that his family's situation was "hopeless," and that he "had nothing to look forward to." But as unfortunate as Derrick's situation was, he also realized that his extreme language was making him feel even worse. Derrick conquered his all-or-nothing thinking by realizing that although his salary reduction would mean having to pinch pennies and cut back on expenses for a while, it didn't mean that life would be a "complete mess." After all, he had a solid marriage and very supportive family and friends. He was also a dedicated and award-winning teacher. Derrick also discovered that his situation wasn't the "hopeless insurmountable disaster" that he'd thought. He was able to make up some of the salary cut by tutoring students privately after school—which he enjoyed very much. When he recognized the shades of gray—life would have *some* challenges, but wouldn't be *completely* awful—Derrick was able to get a better handle on his stress.

Can you see the shades of gray where you fall into the all-or-nothing thinking trap? Fill in the worksheet below with some of your black-and-white cognitions in the left column and challenge yourself to come up with alternative thoughts that include shades of gray.

REVISING BLACK-AND-WHITE THINKING

Black-and-white/All-or-nothing thoughts	Shades-of-gray thinking
Example: *My new sweater has a pull in it—now it's totally ruined.*	*It's not perfect, but one pull doesn't ruin the entire garment. It's wearable, and probably no one but me will even notice the pull.*

Looking for Extremist Language

Another way to challenge all-or-nothing thinking is to begin noticing particular words and phrases that refer to extremes, such as *always, never, everyone, no one, everything, nothing, every, completely, totally, absolutely, perfect,* and the like. Even though we often think (and say) things like "*Everyone* knows how to change a flat tire," "He *always* tries to push his political views on me," and "My mother can't do *anything* right!" these ideas are unrealistic exaggerations. If you notice them in your own repertoire, work hard not to use them. And replace them with more flexible terms such as *often, rarely, usually, most, almost, the majority, many, nearly,* and so on.

You can also challenge your thinking by asking yourself rhetorical questions such as "Is it really true that *everyone* else in the world can change a flat tire?" "Does he really *always* try to push his political views on me, or am I exaggerating?" and "Is there really *absolutely nothing* (not one thing at all) that Mother can do right?"

When you challenge your all-or-nothing thinking this way, you'll usually (but not *always!*) find that the extremes don't apply. In fact, if you can think of even a single example that contradicts the all-or-nothing belief, you've logically proven the belief wrong and can replace it with more flexible and logical thinking. For example, while *many* people know how to change flat tires, certainly not *everyone* does. And that relative of yours might *often* try to push his political views on you, but there are probably times when he hasn't. Finally, while there are *some* things that Mother might not do very well, you can likely find other things that she does do well.

Vince was a terrific college basketball player with realistic hopes of making it to the pros one day. Yet despite being outstanding in most aspects of the game, he felt overwhelming anxiety about making foul shots. When Vince practiced in the gym, away from the big crowds and bright lights, he could make over 80% of his shots; but it was another story when he was in the arena playing in real games and under real pressure to perform well. "I *never* make foul shots," Vince said. "I'll *never* get over this problem and *never* make it to the NBA."

Using the strategies you've just read about, how would Vince change his all-or-nothing thinking? In the following spaces, write in more adaptive and realistic thoughts that would help Vince reduce his stress:

_____

_____

_____

_____

If you suggested Vince think alternative cognitions such as "I'm having trouble with foul shots in games, but not in practice, so I know I can do this" and "I play very well in other areas of the game besides foul shooting," then you've got it—you're ready to challenge your own black-and-white thinking. These alternative thoughts are every bit as logical as they are less stress-provoking—and remember, using logic is the key. If Vince could see things in this light, he'd take some of the pressure off himself, feel more comfortable at the foul line, and probably make more shots.

Musturbation (Demandingness)

We all have our own ideals when it comes to how to live life and how we'd prefer people treat us. In our society, succeeding at work or school, having nice things, being attractive, popular, and self-disciplined are all highly valued. And because we want others to like and accept us, we strive for these ideals. In general, there's nothing wrong with that. In fact, it's healthy to want to succeed. Being outgoing and friendly, for example, helps you develop strong relationships, which keep stress at bay. But when you hold on to these ideals and preferences in a rigid and inflexible way—as if they're rules or demands from on high—you cause yourself a great deal of stress, especially when you can't meet your own expectations or when things are beyond your control. In cognitive therapy, we call these rules and demands *musts* or *shoulds*. If, for example, you sometimes feel shy and self-conscious, yet you tell yourself, "I *must* feel confident and relaxed," you'll end up very stressed and unhappy.

It's the same with making demands on other people. The truth is, we can't control their behavior; and unfortunately they sometimes let us down. But while it's reasonable to feel disappointed or annoyed with others when this happens, it's unreasonable to hold people to certain standards for how you feel they *must* or *should* act ("He *should* have returned my call"; "People *must* respect me"). When you do this, you find yourself feeling angry and resentful toward others when inevitably things don't go the way you want. And in the end, this is a waste of your energy because anger, grudges, and blame don't solve any problems. They just stress you out.

Here are some common *musts* and *shoulds* that many people with stress demand of themselves and others. Put a check next to any of these traps that you fall into.

Demands on Yourself

❏ I must be liked and approved of by everyone.

❏ I must always be successful in the things I do.

❏ I should always do things perfectly.

❏ I should be attractive (thin, muscular, sexy, and so on).

❏ I should have a boyfriend, girlfriend, or spouse/partner.

❏ I should always feel confident.

❏ I must be clear about my future and know where I'm heading.

❏ I should say the right things at the right time.

❏ I must be able to meet other people's expectations.

❏ I should never make mistakes.

Demands on Other People

❏ People should always be respectful.

❏ Others must follow the rules.

❏ People should see things the way I see them.

❏ People should help others in need.

❏ People should treat me fairly.

❏ People must not get in the way of my attaining my goals.

You might be thinking, "What's this? You're asking me to give up on my goals and ideals and settle for something less?" Actually, not at all. While it's all well and good to *prefer* that things be a certain way, it's also common sense that you can't always get what you want. The trouble with *musts* and *shoulds* is that you're demanding to get what you want, as if by some absolute decree or commandment. But it's not a mandate—it's your *preference*. When things don't go your way, you have choices. You can try to achieve what you want, but be flexible and accept that some things don't go as you wish, or you can "*must*urbate" and continue to stubbornly insist that they do go your way. The first option is healthy and logical. It leads to being adaptable, agreeable, and stress free. If *musts* and *shoulds* dominate your thinking, however, you're likely to end up stressed, miserable, and (ironically) less effective at coping with the situation. Here are some strategies for challenging your own *must*urbation thinking.

Turning <u>Shoulds</u> and <u>Musts</u> into Preferences

A straightforward way of challenging *shoulds* and *musts* is to rethink them as *preferences*, *wishes*, and *desires*—rather than rigid rules or demands. When you're feeling very angry or frustrated, try to identify the rule that's been broken. Did someone (perhaps even yourself) behave as you feel he or she *shouldn't*? Maybe things didn't go as you feel they *must*. When you're frustrated or angry, look for these sorts of thoughts and write them in the worksheet on the next page. Then challenge your thinking by reminding yourself that these aren't absolutes, but rather *preferences*. Convert the *musts* to healthier, more flexible cognitions as in the example in the worksheet.

Josh's tailor promised that Josh's new suit would be altered and ready to wear for his job interview on Thursday. But when Josh went to pick up the suit on Wednesday, the tailor apologized and said it wouldn't be ready until the following week. Josh got angry and very stressed. "I absolutely *must* have the new suit for my interview," he told himself. His other automatic thoughts were "The tailor should have had it done on time" and

---

EYE PENER

Conditional versus Unconditional *Musts* and *Shoulds*

Some types of *musts* and *shoulds* can be sensible and realistic under certain conditions—and they're called *conditional musts* and *shoulds*. You can spot them because they'll usually contain the word *if*. For example, "*If* you are going to drive your car, you *must* have gasoline in the fuel tank"; and "You *should* work hard *if* you want to get a promotion." *Unconditional musts* and *shoulds*, however, are unrealistic because they're absolutistic—there are no *ifs*. For example, "You absolutely *must* have gasoline in your car"; "You *should* work hard under all circumstances"; and "I positively *must* get a promotion." It's these *unconditional musts*, *shoulds*, and other demands that cause so much stress in your life.

CONVERTING RIGID THINKING TO FLEXIBLE THINKING

Rigid thinking: *Musts*, *shoulds*, and other rules	Flexible thinking: Preferences
Example: *If I do something to help Shelley, she should return the favor and do something to help me.*	*It would be nice—and I'd <u>prefer</u> it—if Shelley returned my favor, but there's no rule that says she <u>should</u> or <u>must</u>. I can't control Shelley's behavior.*

"People should do what they say they're going to do!" These cognitions led to extreme stress—but what could Josh really do?

Sometimes we're at the mercy of others—and they don't always come through for us. Rather than get angry and stressed—which doesn't solve any problems and only makes matters worse—you'll want to use cognitive therapy to reframe how you look at the situation. Being able to step back and recognize that your demands are really preferences in disguise is an extremely useful tool for managing stress. Think about some less stressful thoughts that might have been helpful for Josh in this situation. Write them in the following spaces:

_____

_____

_____

Hopefully you came up with alternative thoughts such as *I'd prefer* to have the new suit to wear for the interview, but I guess I'll have to wear an older one; I wish the tailor had stuck to his word, but I can't really control what he does. These types of thoughts would help Josh control his stress. Sure, he'd be annoyed (3 or 4 out of 10 on the rating scale), but in the end, what could he do about it now?

Challenging the Logic of <u>Musturbation</u>

Turning some demands into preferences might be easier said than done, especially when it comes to "big-ticket" *musts* such as "I [or my children] *must* get good grades in school," "Children *must* respect their elders," and "I *must* succeed in my job." You might feel that these really *are* imperatives—much too important to consider mere *preferences*. But when you look at it logically, even these seemingly urgent *musts* are really desires and preferences—perhaps very strong preferences. And don't take this as diminishing the importance of things like good grades, respecting one's elders, and job success. They're certainly important. But they're not things we can demand unconditionally.

Still don't believe me? Let's consider the logic of some "big-ticket" *musts*. Take job success. Why *must* you succeed in your work? Oh, there are plenty of good reasons that it's *preferable* to succeed: climbing the corporate ladder, earning more money, gaining prestige—you can probably come up with others. But are there any *laws* stating that you *must* succeed? No, there aren't. And that's because success (in work, school, and everything else) isn't an imperative. It's a preference—better than the alternative (failure), but not a law of the universe. The same goes for things like children's respectful behavior toward adults, being in love, and even leading a happy life. You'll actually be less stressed when you give up stubbornly demanding these sorts of things and start accepting that they're your desires—not commandments. Work your hardest and try to achieve your goals, but also keep in mind that there are no laws that things *must* work out as you want them to.

So, a strategy for challenging "big-ticket" *musts* and *shoulds* is to examine the logic in these cognitions. The best way to do that is to ask yourself questions about the *should* or *must* statement, such as the following:

What goes up *must* come down. *Now, **that's** a universal law (the law of gravity). Have you created the illusion for yourself that your wishes and preferences are as fundamental as the natural laws of the universe?*

- "Where's the evidence that he certainly *must* [or *should*] . . . ?"

- "Can I prove that she [or I] positively *should* or *must* . . . ?"

- "Is there a law of the universe that states that people absolutely *must* . . . ?"

- "Where is it written that I *should* . . . ?"

- "Am I confusing what I think absolutely *must* or *should* happen with what I'd *prefer* to happen?"

In addition, you can consider the ill effects of thinking in these terms by asking yourself the following questions:

- "Where does it ultimately get me to demand such things?"

- "What are the pros and cons of demanding that things work out this way versus accepting that although I'd like them to work out, they might not?"

- "As long as I try to demand this, how will I feel?"

- "What does holding this demand do to my stress level—does it increase or decrease it?"

Dean had an anger problem. He'd explode whenever his 9-year-old twins broke his rules. If the boys spoke during worship services, he scolded them on the spot. If they didn't clean their plates at mealtime, he launched into a tirade about not wasting food. Back-talking and jumping on the furniture were what irritated Dean the most. He'd yell so loud the neighbors could hear. Dean strongly believed that children *must* show respect for their parents and obey orders. But Dean was becoming more and more stressed. That's when he tried challenging his demands that his sons behave perfectly: "Where is it written that my kids *must* behave perfectly all the time? Why *should* my boys be any different from other boys? What good does it do to *demand* perfect behavior all the time when I can't control everything they do?" When Dean really considered these questions, he recognized that "boys will be boys," and instead of insisting on flawless behavior, he viewed it as *his preference*. And because it was important to Dean (but not a *dire necessity*) that his boys learn to behave better, he read books on parenting strategies and began applying contingencies for their good (rewards) and bad (punishments) behavior. This helped Dean control his stress and anger; and although his sons weren't perfectly behaved all the time, he was better able to keep his stress level under control when they misbehaved.

Now you try challenging your *musts* and *shoulds* using the questions in the lists above. In the worksheet on the facing page, enter your *must*urbatory cognitions, challenge questions, and more flexible alternative cognitions.

Jumping to Conclusions

When you're stressed and don't know exactly how a situation will turn out, the tendency is to make a prediction—usually a negative one—and then assume it's a foregone conclusion. You might even look for evidence that backs up your prediction and ignore facts that don't. For example, the boss gives you a strange look and you jump to the conclusion that you're being fired. Then you look for more ominous signs (the office seems especially quiet, a coworker goes to lunch without inviting you), but totally overlook the fantastic performance review you got last week! "Fortune-telling" is when you think you know how things will turn out in the future and accept your prediction as fact.

REPLACING *MUSTS* AND *SHOULDS*

Musturbation cognitions	Challenge questions	Flexible alternative cognitions
Example: My son <u>must</u> get into an Ivy League college.	Where is it written that he <u>must</u>? Can I prove this? As long as I demand this, how will I feel?	There's no law that he must go to an Ivy league school; I just <u>want</u> it very much. By <u>demanding</u> it, I only stress myself out because it's not something I can totally control.

"Mind reading" is a form of jumping to conclusions where you believe you know what other people are thinking—usually without even talking to them. The best way to challenge and modify these kinds of stress-inducing cognitions is to step back and carefully examine the evidence for and against them. Here's how.

Examining the Evidence

Carrie's relationship with Mike was getting serious—they'd been together for 3 years. But Carrie was turning 30 and was stressed over why Mike hadn't popped the question. "Maybe he doesn't want to marry me," she told herself when the couple took a ski trip together and there was no proposal. Carrie convinced herself that Mike had found something about her that he didn't like. "Why doesn't he compliment my looks like he used to?" she asked herself. "Maybe he's not attracted to me anymore," she thought. Of course, Carrie's friends couldn't understand all her stress—why would Mike spend so much time with Carrie and take her on a vacation if he didn't love her? Her friends tried to help Carrie see things logically, but Carrie's mind was made up: she was certain Mike was going to dump her soon.

An important step toward managing stress is recognizing that *feeling* anxious and stressed out doesn't necessarily mean your worries are realistic. So, rather than simply assuming the worst-case scenario, it's better to treat your beliefs and interpretations (your B's about the situation) as *guesses* or *hypotheses* as a scientist might do. A scientist who comes up with a hypothesis collects data—factual evidence—to test whether it holds up. By examining the evidence, you'll learn how to consider evidence to help you get a better sense of whether your concerns are realistic and whether there might be alternative (and more realistic) ways of thinking about the situations and thoughts that trigger your stress. In Carrie's case, the evidence strongly suggested that her relationship with Mike was going strong. In other words, she didn't need to stress out or brace for a breakup.

Instead of assuming your negative thought is true, examine the evidence for it.

Collecting and examining this evidence is harder than you might think. That's because stress makes you focus more strongly on evidence that *confirms* your fears and makes you ignore or discount evidence to the contrary. The more stressed out you are, the more this will be the case. Carrie ignored many signs that her relationship was solid (Mike brought her flowers, helped her shop for clothes, and so on) and focused instead on one instance when she had her hopes up that Mike would propose to her. When it didn't happen, she made herself believe this was the end, without even discussing her feelings with Mike. In fact, she believed it so strongly that it overshadowed other, more persuasive evidence to the contrary. To avoid this trap and get a fair and balanced perspective on your stressful events, get into the habit of asking yourself the key questions in the box at the top of the facing page. You might even write them on an index card, which you can then carry around in your pocket or wallet as a reminder.

Key Questions to Help You Examine the Evidence for Your Sources of Stress

- "What does my past experience tell me about this?"

- "What have other people's experiences been?"

- "Have there been times when I expected something bad to happen, but it didn't?"

- "How might someone else look at this situation?"

- "What would I say to a friend about this if the roles were reversed?"

- "Am I confusing a *high*-probability event with a *low*-probability event?"

The process of examining the evidence involves four basic steps:

1. Identify when you're jumping to conclusions over something you're not sure about.
2. Challenge your thoughts by asking yourself the key questions.
3. Weigh the evidence supporting and contradicting these cognitions.
4. Come up with a more realistic belief that's based on the evidence.

I've provided a worksheet (on page 167) to help you work through these four steps. Make copies of it and keep them handy, because jumping to conclusions is a common response to stress. Carrie's completed worksheet appears on the next page.

Awfulizing

Like making mountains out of molehills, when you're under stress your mind turns *slightly* or *fairly* unpleasant situations into complete and utter *catastrophes*. That's not to belittle your situation—you're obviously facing *some* degree of "badness." But when you notice words like *awful*, *horrible*, and *terrible* creeping into your thoughts, it is a good sign you're awfulizing. For example, "It's *terrible* when my friends don't include me in their plans"; "It's *horrible* to fail an exam"; "Getting a flat tire is *awful*"; "If she broke up with me, I'd be *totally devastated*"; and so on. Another indicator is "*What if?*" thinking. Do you get your stomach in knots thinking about what *could* or *might* go wrong? "*What if* we don't have enough money for . . . ?"; "*What if* I don't get a good night's sleep?"; "*What if* the kids don't make friends?" These thinking patterns all lead to intense stress. Here are some strategies for challenging and changing them.

The Unpleasantness Meter

When stress makes you blow things out of proportion, you can use the Unpleasantness Meter (page 168) to help you get some perspective and cope better. Start by thinking

EXAMINING THE EVIDENCE: CARRIE

1. Identify when you're jumping to conclusions:

   Mike hasn't asked me to marry him yet, and for some reason I'm feeling very worried that he's going to dump me. I'll have wasted 3 years on this relationship. This is jumping to conclusions (fortune telling) because I don't know for sure if this is going to happen.

2. Challenge your thoughts by asking yourself the key questions:

   What does my past experience tell me about this? There have been times that I've worried about things like this, but it's usually a false alarm.

   Have there been times when I expected something bad to happen, but it didn't? Yes, this happens a lot. I tend to jump to conclusions often.

   How might someone else look at this situation? All my friends think I'm crazy for feeling this way. They think that Mike will eventually ask me to marry him.

3. Weigh the evidence supporting and contradicting these cognitions:

   a. *Evidence supporting the conclusions I've jumped to:*

      - *He hasn't asked me to get married.*
      - *He doesn't seem to compliment how I look like he used to when we were first dating.*

   b. *Evidence against the conclusions I've jumped to:*

      - *He does lots of things for me, like takes me on vacations, and spends lots of money on me.*
      - *He tells me that he loves me and doesn't spend time with anyone else but me.*
      - *He doesn't seem any less interested in me.*
      - *He seems just as comfortable around me.*
      - *He sometimes compliments me and tells me that I'm beautiful.*
      - *My friends tell me I have nothing to worry about.*

4. Come up with a more realistic belief that is based on the evidence:

   There's not a lot of evidence that Mike's going to break up with me, but there is a lot of evidence that things are just fine between us. Just because he didn't ask me to marry him when I thought it would be the right time doesn't mean he's never going to do it. Maybe I should talk to him about it rather than trying to read his mind.

about whatever it is that you're stressed over (your "current stressor"). On a scale of 0 (not unpleasant at all) to 100 (absolutely awful), place an X on the line to show how unpleasant this situation or event seemed as it was happening (or was about to happen) to you. Then fill in the table by listing unpleasant things you'd consider "truly awful" (such as natural disasters and mass murders), "very unpleasant" (serious accidents and temporary medical problems), "unpleasant" (disagreements and broken household appliances), or "a little unpleasant" (rainy weather, a stiff neck or headache). When you've written

EXAMINING THE EVIDENCE

1. Identify when you're jumping to conclusions:

2. Challenge your thoughts by asking yourself the key questions:

3. Weigh the evidence supporting and contradicting these cognitions:

   a. *Evidence supporting the conclusions I've jumped to:*

   b. *Evidence against the conclusions I've jumped to:*

4. Come up with a more realistic belief that is based on the evidence:

these events in the table, think back to your own stressful event and consider it in light of these other situations.

Bea and her husband were flying to see their grandson's piano recital when their flight was delayed. Understandably, Bea was very upset—but when she lost control and started crying in front of the airline representatives it was clear she was awfulizing: "Do you realize you're making me miss my grandson's piano recital? This is absolutely horrible!" Bea recognized her awfulizing pattern and used the unpleasantness meter strategy to challenge her thinking. She listed truly awful events, such as tsunamis and terrorist attacks; very unpleasant events, such as needing surgery and having a serious car accident; unpleasant events, such as having a fever and arguing with her husband; and situations that were just a bit unpleasant, such as dropping an egg on the floor and getting a paper cut. This helped Bea see that missing the recital was rather *unpleasant*, but not 101% *awful*. As a result, she was able to handle the situation with less stress. By using this approach, you can do the same when you catch yourself awfulizing.

UNPLEASANTNESS METER

Current stressor: _____

Rate the stressor's unpleasantness on the scale below (put an X on the line):

| 0 | 10 | 20 | 30 | 40 | 50 | 60 | 70 | 80 | 90 | 100 |

Not unpleasant   A little unpleasant   Fairly unpleasant   Very unpleasant   Truly *awful*

Complete the table below by listing a few events and situations that you'd place in under each category:

"Truly awful" situations	"Very unpleasant" situations	"Unpleasant" situations	Situations that are "a little" unpleasant

EYE PENER
Key Questions

Whether you're lying awake at night worrying and asking yourself "What if _____?" or spending valuable awake time preoccupied with something *awful* that *could* happen, here are some questions to ask yourself (and explanations) that will help you challenge your awfulizing thinking and reduce your stress.

- **"How will things seem a week from now? A month from now? A year? Five years?"** Although it's easy to lose sight of it, there's a great deal of truth to the ancient saying "This too shall pass." Indeed, most of what we stress out about is temporary because our lives are in a constant state of flux. Think back to something bad that occurred in your past—something you thought was truly terrible. How long did it take before your pain or anxiety started to subside? Do you have any reason to think this situation will be any different? Answering this key question can really help you keep things in perspective.

- **"What serious injury would I accept in place of this situation?"** Which of these injuries would you rather have than face your stressor? A blister, paper cut, bad sunburn, your finger caught in a car door, broken arm, broken jaw, amputated finger, losing your sight, losing a limb—do I need to go any further? Most people would swap only a minor injury for their stressor—what does that say about its true awfulness?

- **"Is this really so horrible or important that it will affect my entire future?"** This is similar to the first question. The truth is you'd be hard pressed to find too many events or situations that have the ability to really change the course of your life or affect your entire future. But if you mislead yourself into thinking that this will happen, it sure does intensify your stress levels.

- **"What would be the *worst* thing that could happen?"** That's right, go ahead and try to think of the most awful outcome possible. Then go to work using the techniques in this chapter to challenge your assumption. Where's the evidence that this particular result is likely? Would it be 101% awful or some lesser degree of "badness"? How would you cope if this occurred? If you can deal with the *worst possible* outcome, then things might not be truly as horrible as they seem. Congratulations—you have some perspective!

"I-Can't-Stand-Its" (Low Frustration Tolerance)

Stress makes putting up with hassles and irritations even more difficult. But how often have you said to yourself "I can't stand it," and yet you're still alive right now (and sometimes even able to enjoy yourself)? When you repeat this often enough, you start to convince yourself that a situation really is *awful*—"the end of the world." Your fuse is shorter. You act without thinking. You feel even more stress. This is called *low frustration tolerance* (or LFT), and it's characterized by cognitions such as "I can't stand it"; "I can't take this!"; "It's unbearable!"; "This is ridiculous!"; and "I don't have time for this!" But you can increase your patience and raise your frustration tolerance by challenging these types of cognitions. Here's how.

You *Can* Stand It

"I can't stand it" literally means—dictionary definition—that you cannot exist or live in the presence of something. But the fact is that you won't die or go insane from things like waiting in line or getting stuck in traffic, having to deal with difficult people, visiting the dentist, being criticized or embarrassed, working on a challenging project, and the like. You *can* stand it—and what's more, you get to choose *how* you stand it. It might be a matter of semantics, but you can tell yourself that the situation is *unbearable* and be stressed out and frustrated, or you can remind yourself that even though you don't like being in the situation, you can still put up with it. Cognitions such as "This is *unpleasant* (or *inconvenient*), but I can handle it" and "What doesn't kill me makes me stronger" are useful in defeating LFT. Here are some questions to ask yourself to challenge LFT cognitions:

- "Is this truly *unbearable*, or am I exaggerating?"

- "Can I survive in the presence of _____?"

- "Is this really going to *kill* me, or is it something I just really don't like?"

- "Will this cause a heart attack? Will it make me faint? Will it make my eyes pop out of my head?"

- "If I really *can't stand it*, why am I still upright (and even smiling sometimes)?"

- "If it's really *too much* to take, when did I die as a consequence?"

In the worksheet on the facing page, try using these questions to convert your own LFT cognitions into more adaptive, less stressful thinking as in the example.

Labeling

Nature designed the human brain to use shortcuts in order to understand the complex world around us. This helps us solve problems efficiently and keep our problem-solving capacity on call all the time. So, when you're stressed out and someone does something that rubs you the wrong way, the tendency is to assume that the person *always* does this kind of thing because of a personality defect: "She's annoying." "He's a fool." "They're all idiots." You might even do this to yourself: "I'm a loser." "I'm inferior." But this kind

*There's no person who can be defined by a single adjective. Labels are for **behaviors**— not **people**.*

COUNTERING LFT THOUGHTS

LFT cognitions	Less stressful cognitions
Example: *I can't stand my kid's fifth-grade teacher!* She doesn't know how to teach math or how to talk to parents.	*I don't like this situation, but I can put up with it for the rest of the school year. It's not going to kill me or permanently harm my child.*

of shortcut prevents us from seeing people as they really are. When you label *others*, you start to look for behaviors that confirm your negative view (and ignore behaviors that go against your label), and that makes you more stressed. Labeling *yourself* amounts to beating yourself up—a thinking pattern that leads to feeling depressed. Either way, labeling is a glaring oversimplification. How can you short-circuit this stress-inducing shortcut? Read on.

Try to Define the Label

When you label someone else as "a crook" or "a coward," or yourself as "inferior," ask yourself what these labels really mean.

- *What's the definition of a crook?* Wouldn't he or she have to disobey the law 100% of the time? No exceptions? Not even one example of moral or law-abiding behavior? Is there really anyone like that?

- *What's a coward?* Wouldn't this person have to be afraid of absolutely *everything*? Never showing any confidence or bravery whatsoever? Literally never standing up to anyone or anything? Does anyone like that really exist?

- *What does it mean to be an "inferior human being"?* Wouldn't this person have to be far below every other human being in every single way possible?

When you think about it carefully, there's really no such thing as a crook, coward, inferior person, or any other label. That's because everyone—and I mean *everyone*—has his or her own areas of strength and skill and of vulnerability and weakness. People are complex—much too complex to be defined only by their weaknesses. And way too complicated to be described using a single adjective. You'll reduce your stress levels when you take a balanced and logical view of yourself and others as *people* who are capable of doing both good and bad (but who themselves are neither "good" nor "bad") and of having success and failure (but who themselves are neither "successes" nor "failures").

Judge the <u>Behavior</u>, Not the <u>Person</u>

Another way to overcome labeling is to focus on judging people's (or your own) *behavior*, rather than their *personhood*. Remember that everyone (yourself included) makes good and bad decisions, is sometimes brave and sometimes afraid, and sometimes succeeds yet sometimes fails. If Kelly sometimes cheats but sometimes is honest, how can she be a *cheater* (or an honest *person*)? If Dylan is nasty to some people but nice to others, how can he be a nasty *person* (or a nice one, for that matter)? When we label people, we're usually referring to just a sample of their behavior that we like or don't like. But try to stick to labeling the behavior and don't carry it over to the person: "Dylan said something very nasty to his next-door neighbor"; "It was very nice of Dylan to walk his younger sister home from the bus stop." Neither make Dylan a nice or nasty *person*. When you focus on the specifics of the situation, rather than negatively labeling people, you'll start appreciating people for who they are and what they're capable of ("What Don *did* was hypocritical, but that doesn't make Don a *hypocrite*"). When you acknowledge your own personal strengths and weaknesses ("I'm not athletic, but I do other things very well") rather than judging yourself as a person based on your weaknesses ("I'm a loser because I'm not athletic"), you'll reduce your stress. Use the worksheet on the facing page to practice changing your labels into logical and stress-reducing cognitions about people and their behavior.

REPLACING LABELS

Labels	Cognitions that reduce stress
Examples: 1. She's a spoiled brat. 2. I'm such a moron for leaving the door unlocked and causing the house to be burglarized.	1. Her parents often pamper her. 2. I was careless, and it led to someone burglarizing the house. This doesn't make me a moron—everyone makes mistakes. This was an especially costly one.

9

Relaxing Your Body
and Clearing Your Mind

Being able to relax, unwind, and clear your mind will make you more successful at defusing the stress that you already feel and help you prevent stress from occurring in the first place. But if you're chronically stressed out, you're probably having trouble doing so. Maybe you've even "forgotten" how to relax. Does it seem like you *can't* clear your mind of racing stressful thoughts? That's why I've included this chapter on relaxation and meditation strategies. These techniques affect your brain and body to directly counteract the damaging physical and mental effects of stress and help you achieve states of deep rest and mental clarity. What's more, when you're relaxed and thinking clearly, you'll be able to use the other techniques in this workbook even more successfully. And last but not least, the skills you'll learn to use in this chapter can improve your overall health and well-being. Researchers have found that learning to relax and meditate is associated with the following important health and lifestyle benefits:

- Relief from aches and pains

- Relief from generalized anxiety disorder

- Reduced depression

- Better sleep

- Increased daily energy (reduced tiredness and fatigue)

- Increased motivation

- Increased productivity

- Better decision-making ability

- Lower blood pressure

- Reduced irritability

- Strengthened immune system

Although relaxation and meditation are each important parts of stress management, they reduce stress in different ways. Learning to relax brings your body back into balance when it's affected by stress: deepening your breathing, reducing stress hormones, slowing down your heart rate and blood pressure, and relaxing your muscles. With relaxation, you're directly reducing the physical signs and symptoms of stress. Meditation, on the other hand, helps you achieve a sense of mental balance that translates to feeling more stable in all your activities. Rather than relax you, it helps you develop a healthier relationship to the physical signs of stress. In the process it might also relax you, but that is not its goal. And best of all, with a little practice, you can reap the benefits of these techniques. You'll learn the basics of meditation later on in this chapter. To begin with, though, we'll focus on two techniques—diaphragmatic breathing and muscle relaxation—to help you use your body's relaxation response to manage your stress.

THE RELAXATION RESPONSE

The relaxation response is your body's ability to get you physically relaxed and mentally alert. It involves a release of neurotransmitters and other chemicals that signal your brain to tell your body's muscles and organs to ease up—basically the opposite of the fight-or-flight response. When this happens, more blood flows to your brain, which causes alertness and helps you think more clearly. But if you experience lots of stress, your body might not be able to achieve this response very easily on its own. The good news, though, is that you can learn how to achieve relaxation using a variety of techniques, such as:

- Deep breathing

- Progressive muscle relaxation

- Mindfulness meditation

- Yoga

- Biofeedback

- Visual imagery

*The relaxation response is **not** lazily lying (or sleeping) around the house. It's a special kind of mental activity that leaves the body relaxed. It's something that takes practice to learn; and it's best practiced while you're awake.*

Which of these techniques are the best for triggering your relaxation response? Researchers have found that in general they're all equally effective at helping you calm down your body and mind. But different people tend to prefer different techniques, and they tend to practice their preferred ones most, which naturally produces the greatest benefit. Because research shows that deep breathing, progressive muscle relaxation, and mindfulness meditation are the easiest and most preferred relaxation methods, I've included them in this chapter.

BREATHING TECHNIQUES

Believe it or not, there are different ways to breathe—some more effective than others. And poor breathing habits can contribute to stress and cause a host of unpleasant physical symptoms. If you habitually breathe the way you "take a deep breath" at your doctor's direction during a physical exam, you're using *chest (thoracic) breathing*, expanding your chest and raising your shoulders to suck in air as you inhale. Chest breathing is too quick and too shallow. It reduces the amount of oxygen you take in and in turn reduces the amount that reaches your brain and other organs. This causes temporary sensations such as shortness of breath, feelings of fatigue, lightheadedness, numbness and tingling, agitation, and confusion—and thus perpetuates the stress cycle. You may be aware of breathing this way, noticing that you're often hyperventilating and feeling short of breath. But if you're under a great deal of stress, you're probably not paying too much attention to how you breathe and may have been breathing this way out of habit, exacerbating your stress, for a long time.

EYE OPENER

Benefits of Diaphragmatic Breathing

Making abdominal or diaphragmatic breathing (described on the facing page) a habit will benefit your body in numerous ways that go beyond stress management. Here are a few:

- Oxygenation of your blood
- Facilitation of the removal of waste products from your body's organs, including the brain
- Massaging of the internal organs by the diaphragm
- Promotion of relaxation and health
- Boosts in mental functioning
- Provision of a simple and easy relaxation technique that you can do just about anywhere
- Reversal of the stress response

Just five minutes of diaphragmatic breathing is a helpful start to promote health, short-circuit stress, and combat any effects of shallow breathing.

In contrast, *abdominal or diaphragmatic breathing* is the most natural type of breathing, in which the abdomen expands outward with each breath, making room for the diaphragm—the muscle dividing your belly from your lungs—to contract and draw air deep into the lungs. (If you can't picture it, watch a baby, or even an adult, breathe while sleeping.) When you exhale, the abdomen and diaphragm relax. It's deeper, slower, more rhythmic, and more relaxing than breathing with your chest. Diaphragmatic breathing ensures that your muscles and organs—including your brain—have an adequate supply of oxygen, normalizes the body's production of energy, and improves the removal of carbon dioxide and other waste products from your body. When you become more conscious of your own breathing habits and practice more abdominal breathing, you'll balance the levels of oxygen and carbon dioxide in your body, normalize your heart rate, and reduce the muscle tension associated with stress. When your body functions at this high rate of efficiency, your brain gets the oxygen and nutrients it needs (and its waste products removed effectively), so your ability to think clearly is also boosted. Diaphragmatic breathing is one of the best ways to bring about the relaxation response.

Learning and Practicing Diaphragmatic Breathing

Diaphragmatic breathing is one of the best ways to lower stress in the body and clear your mind, and it can be used just about anywhere. Breathing deeply sends a message to your brain to calm down and relax. The brain then sends this message to your body. The physical signs of stress, such as increased heart rate, muscle tension, and high blood pressure, all decrease as you breathe this way. And when your body isn't using up so much oxygen to keep your stress response racing along, more of it reaches your brain cells, leading to improved mental functioning.

Preparing to Practice

Before you begin, measure your resting breathing rate. Using a watch or a timer, count the number of breaths you take in one minute while you're inactive (such as sitting in a chair or lying in bed). If, like most people, you tend to breathe with your chest, you probably take 10 to 12 breaths per minute. Enter your breathing rate in the space below.

My resting breathing rate = _____ breaths per minute.

Learning Diaphragmatic Breathing

As with learning any other skill, teaching yourself to breathe with your abdomen requires some time and practice. But even if you're not used to breathing this way, the good news is that it won't take very long to learn. Breathing exercises are easy to learn. You can do them whenever you want, and you don't need any special tools or equipment to do them. The goal of the exercise is to breathe deeply from your *stomach* (not from your chest or shoulders), getting as much fresh air as possible in your lungs. Now find a quiet place where you won't be interrupted for at least 15 minutes and follow these steps:

1. Sit comfortably with your back straight. Put one hand on your chest and the other on your stomach.

2. Breathe in through your nose. When you inhale, let your belly expand outward. Think of the air going into your lungs and notice the feeling of your stomach expanding. The hand on your stomach should rise. The hand on your chest should move very little if at all.

3. Exhale through your mouth, pushing out as much air as you can while contracting your abdominal muscles. The hand on your stomach should move in as you exhale, but your other hand should move very little.

4. Continue to breathe in through your nose and out through your mouth. Try to inhale enough so that your lower abdomen rises and falls. Count slowly as you exhale.

5. Some people have difficulty breathing from their abdomen while sitting up. If that's the case for you, try it lying on the couch, bed, or floor. Put a small book on your stomach and try to breathe so that the book rises as you inhale and falls as you exhale. Your chest should not move up and down—just your stomach (and the book).

How to Practice

For the next 2 weeks, try to practice at least three times a day for 10 to 15 minutes in a variety of different situations. Here are some situations in which my own patients practice their deep breathing:

- "When I'm driving to and from work."—Aliza, a talent agent

- "While I'm sitting on the couch, watching TV."—Aron, father of two

- "I can practice diaphragmatic breathing during classes."—Jack, a college student

- "I like to practice while I read or work in my office"—Nina, a college professor

You'll also want to keep track of your stress levels before and after each practice. Use the Diaphragmatic Breathing Practice Log on the facing page to record this information (make extra copies of the form). With practice, you'll be able to automatically take diaphragmatic breaths in stressful situations to relax yourself.

Another way to help you change the habit of chest breathing is to set an alarm for every hour, and when it goes off, check to see which type of breathing technique you're using. Are you breathing diaphragmatically? Great! Are you breathing from your chest? It means you need to keep practicing to kick this habit.

DIAPHRAGMATIC BREATHING PRACTICE LOG

Instructions: Practice diaphragmatic breathing for 10 to 15 minutes three times each day for 2 weeks. Enter the date, time, and situation in which you complete each practice. Rate your stress level before and after each practice from 0 (no stress) to 10 (extremely stressed).

Week # _____

Date	Time	Place/situation	Beginning stress level (0 to 10)	Ending stress level (0 to 10)

PROGRESSIVE MUSCLE RELAXATION

Progressive muscle relaxation is another effective and widely used strategy for stress relief. It's based on the fact that tensing and relaxing your muscles activates the relaxation response. Everyone has a certain amount of tension in their muscles—even while resting. But if you're under a great deal of stress, you probably have a higher degree of resting tension; and that can be painful and tiring. When you purposely alternate tensing up and then relaxing your muscles, the tension level not only returns to its original levels, but automatically drops *below* the original level, producing even greater relaxation.

The *progressive* part of this relaxation technique refers to moving through your body—starting with your feet—tensing and relaxing the different muscle groups. When you practice this technique repeatedly, it helps you learn what tension—as well as complete relaxation—feels like in different parts of the body. And this awareness helps you become more aware of—and counter—the signs of the muscle tension associated with stress. As your body relaxes, so will your mind.

You can start your progressive muscle relaxation exercises with a few minutes of diaphragmatic breathing for an additional level of stress relief.

Learning and Practicing Progressive Muscle Relaxation

Preparing to Practice

Finding a suitable environment for practicing relaxation is important: The ideal location is a dimly lit and quiet place where you can be alone for a little while. Begin by getting comfortable either seated or lying down on your back. Take off your shoes and loosen any tight clothes. Make sure your body is well supported. If you're sitting, use good posture—shoulders back and arms in your lap. You can either close your eyes or keep them open (although most people prefer to keep them shut), but if you're wearing glasses, consider removing them. Be sure not to fall asleep! In fact, you want to be somewhat alert. Remain aware of your body and mind, but don't let your mind work too hard. If a stray thought comes along that distracts you, just allow the thought to come and go. Don't try to force it out of your mind.

As you carry out this sequence of exercises, you'll tense different muscle groups above their normal level of tension. You don't need to make it painful—about 5 seconds of tensing is plenty. You'll focus on how the tension feels and then let it go and focus on the sensations of relaxation. Keep your breathing regular (using diaphragmatic breathing) throughout the exercise.

Learning Progressive Muscle Relaxation

1. Begin with about 30 seconds of diaphragmatic breathing as you feel yourself becoming more and more relaxed.

2. Focus on the specific muscle groups described next. At each step, you'll tense and then relax them:

- **Feet and calves:** Focus your attention on your feet and calves. Flex your feet by pulling your toes up toward your knees. Contract your calf muscle and other muscles of your lower legs. Feel the tension build and hold it for 5 seconds. Take a deep breath. As you exhale, say the word "relax" and let the tension go. Take about 20 seconds to notice (and pay close attention to) the difference between the tenseness and feelings of relaxation in your leg muscles.

- **Knees and thighs:** Now bring your attention to your knees and thighs. Straighten your knees and squeeze your legs together. Contract your thigh muscles and all the muscles in your legs. Feel the tension build and hold it for 5 seconds. Take a deep breath. As you exhale, say the word "relax" and let the tension go. Take about 20 seconds to notice (and pay close attention to) the difference between the tenseness and feelings of relaxation in your upper legs.

- **Hips and buttocks:** Next, pay attention to your hips and buttocks. Tense your buttocks by squeezing these muscles inward. Feel the tension build and hold it for 5 seconds. Take a deep breath. As you exhale, say the word "relax" and let the tension go. Take about 20 seconds to notice (and pay close attention to) the difference between the tenseness and feelings of relaxation in your hips and buttocks.

- **Stomach:** Pay attention to your stomach rising and falling with each breath. Inhale and tense your stomach by trying to pull your belly button toward your spine. Tense your abdominal (stomach) muscles. Feel the tension build and hold it for 5 seconds. Take a deep breath. As you exhale, say the word "relax" and let the tension go. Take about 20 seconds to notice (and pay close attention to) the difference between the tenseness and feelings of relaxation in your stomach and abdomen.

- **Upper back:** Focus your attention on the upper part of your back. Try to bring your shoulder blades together to the midline of your back. Tense the muscles in your open back. Feel the tension build and hold it for 5 seconds. Take a deep breath. As you exhale, say the word "relax" and let the tension go. Take about 20 seconds to notice (and pay close attention to) the difference between the tenseness and feelings of relaxation in the muscles of your upper back.

- **Arms and hands:** Next, concentrate on your arms and hands. Turn your hands so your palms are facing down and make two tight fists. Raise and stretch both arms with fists clenched tightly. Feel the tension build and hold it for 5 seconds. Take a deep breath. As you exhale, say the word "relax" and let the tension go. Take about 20 seconds to notice (and pay close attention to) the difference between the tenseness and feelings of relaxation in your hands and arms.

- **Chin, neck, and shoulders:** Now focus on your chin, neck, and shoulders. Bring your chin down toward your chest and raise your shoulders up toward your ears. Feel the tension build and hold it for 5 seconds. Take a deep breath. As you exhale, say the word "relax" and let the tension go. Take about 20 seconds to notice (and pay close attention to) the difference between the tenseness and feelings of relaxation in your neck and shoulder area.

- **Jaw and facial muscles:** Notice the feelings in your face. Clench your teeth together and clench the muscles in the back of your jaw. Turn the corners of your mouth into a tight smile. Wrinkle your nose and squeeze your eyes shut. Tense all facial muscles in toward the center of your face. Feel the tension build and hold it for 5 seconds. Take a deep breath. As you exhale, say the word "relax" and let the tension go. Take about 20 seconds to notice (and pay close attention to) the difference between the tenseness and feelings of relaxation in your face.

- **Forehead:** Finally, focus your attention on your forehead. Raise your eyebrows and tense the muscles across your forehead. Feel the tension build and hold it for 5 seconds. Take a deep breath. As you exhale, say the word "relax" and let the tension go. Take about 20 seconds to notice (and pay close attention to) the difference between the tenseness and feelings of relaxation in your forehead.

3. End the exercise as follows: Focus on the feelings of relaxation over your entire body—from your head, over your face, through your shoulders and down your back, down through your arms and hands, over your chest and stomach, flowing through your hips and buttocks, into your thighs, knees, and calves, and finally into your ankles and feet. Continue your diaphragmatic breathing for a few minutes. Then count backwards from 10 to 1. As you do so, gradually become more aware of your surroundings, stretch your arms, legs, and head, and open your eyes. Slowly rise from your sitting or lying position feeling energized, refreshed, and relaxed.

How to Practice

If you don't feel much of a difference the first time you do progressive relaxation, don't worry—it's normal. In fact, it might take going through the sequence of tensing and relaxing several times before you really notice the benefits and begin to enjoy it. Some people even find practicing relaxation to be *stressful* at first. You might notice "side effects" such as tingling feelings or restlessness. This is also normal and not a sign that you're doing something wrong or that the technique won't work for you. As you practice and become more familiar with the exercises, they'll help you relax more deeply and the side effects will fade away. You'll eventually be able to use them to relax in more hectic situations, which will help you view those situations as less threatening and stressful. Just keep in mind that it will probably take several tries before you really get the hang of it. Stick with it.

Once you've gone through the exercises a few times and are familiar with the sequence of body parts, you'll want to practice so that it becomes more and more routine. I suggest that over the next 2 weeks you practice progressive muscle relaxation at least once a day under the same private and quiet conditions. As with diaphragmatic breathing, you'll also want to keep track of how much your stress level goes down with each practice. Use the Progressive Muscle Relaxation Practice Log on the next page to record this information (make extra copies of the form). After practicing this technique for 2 weeks, you might want to move on to the shortened version, which I describe in the next section.

A Shortened Relaxation Sequence

The following shortened version of progressive muscle relaxation is a good way to use the technique in all kinds of situations when you may not have time for the full routine. The shortened form reduces the nine muscle groups to four groups:

1. Legs, feet, and buttocks

2. Back and stomach

3. Arms, shoulders, and neck

4. Face

Another name for this short version is "cue-controlled relaxation" because each time you let the tension go, you also practice saying a *cue word* (or phrase), such as "calm" or "let it go" to yourself. Doing this helps you associate the cue word with feelings of relaxation, so that eventually the cue word alone produces a relaxed state. Here are some suggestions for cue words and phrases—feel free to come up with your own:

- "Relax."

- "Calm."

- "Let it go."

- "Peace."

- "Still."

- "Serenity now."

When you practice cue-controlled relaxation, start in the same environment where you practiced the longer version. After about a week of twice daily practice, you'll be ready to practice it in other situations and with potential distractions. Here's what to practice:

PROGRESSIVE MUSCLE RELAXATION PRACTICE LOG

Instructions: Practice progressive muscle relaxation once every day for two weeks. Enter the date and time you complete each practice. Rate your stress level before and after each practice from 0 (no stress) to 10 (extremely stressed).

Date	Time	Stress level before (0 to 10)	Stress level after (0 to 10)

- **Group 1—Legs, feet, and buttocks:** Straighten and tense all the muscles in both of your legs. Pull your toes up toward your knees. Inhale slowly (using diaphragmatic breathing) as you apply and hold the tension. Hold it for 8 to 10 seconds and then, as you let go of the tension, exhale slowly and say your cue word to yourself. Relax for 15 to 20 seconds.

- **Group 2—Stomach and back:** Take a deep breath and suck in your stomach as hard as possible for 8 to 10 seconds. Inhale slowly (using diaphragmatic breathing) as you apply and hold the tension. Hold it for 8 to 10 seconds and then, as you let go of the tension, exhale slowly and say your cue word to yourself. Relax for 15 to 20 seconds.

- **Group 3—Arms, shoulders, and neck:** Fold your arms across your chest and make fists with both of your hands. Tense the muscles in your arms, fists, and shoulders. Inhale slowly (using diaphragmatic breathing) as you apply and hold the tension. Hold it for 8 to 10 seconds and then, as you let go of the tension, exhale slowly and say your cue word to yourself. Then relax for 15 to 20 seconds.

- **Group 4—Face:** Tense your facial muscles by wrinkling your forehead and pursing your lips. Inhale slowly (using diaphragmatic breathing) as you apply and hold the tension. Hold it for 8 to 10 seconds and then, as you let go of the tension, exhale slowly and say your cue word to yourself. Focus on the feelings of relaxation over your whole body—from your head, over your face, through your shoulders and down your back, down through your arms and hands, over your chest and stomach, flowing through your hips and buttocks, into your thighs, knees, and calves, and finally into your ankles and feet. Continue your diaphragmatic breathing for a few minutes. Then count backward from 10 to 1. As you count, gradually become more aware of your surroundings, stretch your arms, legs, and head, and open your eyes.

The Cue-Controlled Relaxation Practice Log on the next page is where you can keep track of your practice with this technique (make extra copies of the form). For the first week, practice in a comfortable and quiet place. Then, for the second week, try it in different situations where you might be distracted, such as at work, while driving, or while waiting in line at the store. When you feel you've got it down pat, use this technique anywhere you're feeling stressed to achieve relaxation and stress relief. Here are some examples of situations that my patients have told me they've found using cue-controlled relaxation helpful:

- "Sitting in traffic when I'm going to be late."—Tom, a corporate executive

- "When I'm babysitting and the kids won't listen to me."—Jesse, a babysitter

- "When I'm stressed out about an assignment that I'm working on."—Sharon, a student

CUE-CONTROLLED RELAXATION PRACTICE LOG

Instructions: Practice cue-controlled relaxation once every day for the first week in a calm, quiet place. Enter the date and time you complete each practice. Rate your stress level before and after each practice from 0 (no stress) to 10 (extremely stressed).

Cue word/phrase: _____

Date	Time	Stress level before (0 to 10)	Stress level after (0 to 10)

For the second week, practice once every day in a different situation. Keep track of where you practice each time.

Date	Time	Situation	Stress level before (0 to 10)	Stress level after (0 to 10)

- "During the game if the team is making bad mistakes and losing."—Shane, a baseball coach

- "When the baby won't stop crying."—Harry, a new father

- "When I'm on the plane, before takeoff."—Doreen, who is afraid of flying

- "Taking Mother to her doctor's appointment and sitting in the waiting room."—Emma, whose mother is very ill

- "During tax season and before meeting with my divorce lawyer."—Jodie, an accountant

- "Right before making a sales presentation to the president of my company."—Robert, a businessman

MEDITATION

Meditation involves centering your attention and your awareness within yourself to clear and focus your mind. Research shows that it can also have beneficial effects on your body, such as lowering blood pressure and reducing pain. It's even been shown to boost your immune system so that you recover more quickly from illnesses such as the flu. There are many different types of meditation. In this chapter you'll learn two that are helpful for reducing stress: *mantra* and *mindfulness* meditation. In mantra meditation, you repeat a *mantra*—a word or phrase that has significance for you—to help you clear your mind. Mindfulness involves learning to stay in the present moment rather than dwelling on the past or future. Both meditation styles involve a passive, nonjudgmental attitude. That is, you work on treating your thoughts as if they're just leaves on a stream floating past you. You don't engage them, fight them, or hold on to them. You simply allow them to come and go through your mind. This is beneficial because it helps you focus on the present moment rather than reliving the past or preliving the future.

Mantra Meditation

In mantra meditation, you repeat (either aloud or to yourself) a syllable, word, or phrase (the *mantra*) that's soothing and that has meaning for you. When you meditate, this is what you focus your mind on. Repeating the mantra helps center your attention and bring you back when your mind temporarily drifts away.

What Mantra Should I Use?

Choosing a mantra isn't hard. Just find a syllable (such as "om"), a word (such as "peace" or "shalom"), or even a short phrase (such as "clear mind"). When you've got your mantra, write it down in the space at the top of the next page:

My meditation mantra: _____

Stick with your mantra through your entire meditation practice. The goal is to have it become connected with the experience of meditating.

How to Practice

Begin by getting into the "meditation position"—sitting (or lying) in a comfortable chair or on a cushion on the floor or ground. Use good posture: back straight, upper body balanced on your hips, chin down, and mouth closed. Your eyes can either be open or closed. Make sure your shoulders aren't shrugged up toward your ears—bring them down as low as they'll go. Your hands can be in your lap or on your knees and should feel rested. The main thing is that you should feel no muscle tension when you meditate. Next, follow these steps:

1. Using diaphragmatic breathing, take some slow deep breaths. Bring your attention to your body, right then, and right there, and pay attention to your "in breath" and your "out breath." Focus on your breaths. Feel each one from all the way down in your stomach. Let yourself ease into a regular and even breathing pattern. And just breathe away any thoughts, ideas, or images that might be distracting or upsetting to you.

2. Do you have any tension left in your body? Take a moment to scan for it, and if you find any, let it go. Then turn your attention back to your breathing.

3. Now begin repeating your mantra over and over, at regular intervals (either to yourself or softly aloud), but slowly. Let it find its own pace and rhythm; don't try to force it. Stay focused on your mantra. If you notice any distracting thoughts or sensations in your body, just observe them and then return your attention to your mantra. Continue repeating your mantra for 20 minutes at first, building up to 45 minutes once or twice a day. Remain in this state for as long as you'd like.

4. When you're ready to end your meditation session, take a deep breath, exhale fully, and open your eyes, if they were closed during your meditation. You can say to yourself, "I'm refreshed and alert."

As with any other skill, regular practice is a must if you want to get the full benefits of mantra meditation. As you work at it, you'll notice that you get better at quieting your mind and focusing on your mantra. You'll get more skilled at just *experiencing* thoughts and internal sensations without *reacting* to them (which you'll also learn in mindfulness meditation). I suggest practicing every day for 2 weeks, even if it's just for 10 minutes at a time. As you get more comfortable with meditation, you can increase your practice time, perhaps to 1 hour or more each day, a few times per week. Keep track of your practicing using the Meditation Practice Log on page 189 (make extra copies of the form).

MEDITATION PRACTICE LOG

Instructions: Practice meditating every day for 2 weeks. Enter the date and time of each practice and the type of meditation you used (mantra, mindfulness, or another form you have learned). Rate your stress level from 0 (no stress) to 10 (extremely stressed) before and after each session.

Date	Time	Type of meditation	Beginning stress level (0 to 10)	Ending stress level (0 to 10)

Mindfulness Meditation

As you've learned, much of your stress is caused by thinking patterns such as jumping to conclusions, catastrophizing, and analyzing thoughts about the future or past. When you meditate, however, your aim is to teach yourself to block out these maladaptive cognitions and get into the present moment, focusing on what you're doing and feeling in the here and now. When you focus on something that calms your mind—breathing, a mantra, or otherwise—your mind enters its own state of calmness.

But when you're stressed, it's hard to simply put these seemingly pressing matters aside. And you might fall into the trap of trying to fight or push them out of your mind. Unfortunately, though, this strategy doesn't work very well. In fact, when you try forcing a thought, image, or feeling out of your mind, it usually comes back . . . sometimes even *stronger* than in the first place. That's where mindfulness meditation comes in. This type of meditation helps you just *experience* and *accept* your thoughts and feelings *as they are* rather than trying to regulate, dismiss, or change them. After all, thoughts and feelings can't hurt you; they're just in your head. They're part of what it means to be human. And just look at this list of some of the benefits that research shows mindfulness meditation can have: increased self-awareness and self-acceptance, decreased anxiety in the face of stressors, increased flexibility and adaptability to change, and better immune system functioning to help your body fight illnesses.

How Do You Deal with Unwanted Thoughts and Feelings?

The following list contains several common ways people respond to unpleasant thoughts, images, and feelings. You'll want to know about these strategies so you can work on stopping them when you meditate. Place a check mark next to each strategy that you use:

❑ Try to reassure yourself about the thought or feeling

❑ Ask others to reassure you about it

❑ Talk yourself through it

❑ Try to figure out the thought's logic

❑ Try to suppress or dismiss the thought or feeling

❑ Try to avoid thinking about it

❑ Avoid reminders of the thought or feeling

❑ Distract yourself from the thought or feeling by doing something else

❑ Punish yourself for thinking or feeling this way

❑ Tell yourself that you shouldn't think or feel this way

❑ Try to figure out what caused it

When you're stressed out, the way you deal with your stressful thoughts and feelings might be making things worse.

Now consider how these strategies work in the short term and in the long run. Maybe they work temporarily, but do they really help you control the stressful thought or feeling over the long term? Research shows that for most people these strategies are not helpful over the long haul. That's because trying to control, resist, or fight stressful thoughts and feelings just doesn't work—it backfires, sometimes making things worse.

The Mindful Approach to Thoughts and Feelings

There's a story that is often told to explain mindfulness that I first heard while attending a meditation workshop during my work at the Mayo Clinic: Imagine you're throwing a party in your backyard and you've invited lots of friends. But your neighbor, Ted—whom you didn't invite because he's often rude—shows up anyway, starts eating your food, and acts impolitely toward your guests. You ask Ted to leave the party, which he does; and you feel relieved. But a little while later, you notice that Ted has snuck back into the party! So you go get him and throw him out once more. But you see that he's still hanging around just outside the gate to your backyard, threatening to crash your party yet again! What could you do?

One possibility is to stand guard by the gate to make sure he doesn't get back in. But how effective would this strategy be? While it might keep Ted off your yard and out of the party, you'd be missing out on all the fun. You'd be preoccupied with keeping Ted out instead of enjoying your own party.

Another idea would be to lock the gate. But along with keeping Ted out, anyone arriving late that you *did* invite wouldn't be able to get in. And when it's time for your guests to leave, they wouldn't be able to get out. So, locking the gate doesn't seem like it would work very well either.

But since your party is too much fun to miss out on, you could just decide to leave the gate open and go mingle with your friends. And rather than trying so hard to keep Ted out, you could just say to yourself, "If Ted comes in, that's just how it goes." This way, even if Ted does crash the party and starts acting annoyingly, you'll notice that he's there but still enjoy yourself. Sure, it might be better if Ted went home, but at least you're not stuck at the gate missing out on the party. You might even find that when you're not spending so much energy trying to get rid of Ted, you notice some things about him that you hadn't before—maybe he's not as rude as you'd thought; maybe he has a sense of humor. Maybe you can enjoy the party even if you accept that Ted is there.

This story shows you the essence of mindfulness. Ted represents unpleasant thoughts and feelings that you don't want around but that still intrude into your conscious awareness and provoke you to respond by trying to push them away. But as with Ted, trying to resist or fight these thoughts doesn't work. In fact, doing so backfires and keeps you from staying in the moment and enjoying the here and now. What *does* work is just to allow these mental experiences to "happen." You'll find that they're temporary and can't hurt you. Sure, this can feel strange at first since you're so used to trying not to have these thoughts and feelings. But with practice, you can become expert at letting them just come and go. You'll be amazed by how quickly they pass harmlessly out of your mind when you don't try to fight them.

Practicing Mindfulness

When you practice mindfulness meditation, you'll develop a more peaceful relationship with what's happening in the present moment—even if it's stressful thoughts about something in the future, nagging feelings about something that happened in the past, physical discomfort, or external stressors. Here are the steps to follow:

1. Once in your meditation position (described for mantra meditation), begin with diaphragmatic breathing. Focus on your breaths and let yourself ease into a regular breathing pattern. Feel your belly rise and fall as the air enters your nose and leaves through your mouth. Pay attention to how each breath feels.

2. Then try to set aside all thoughts about the past and the future . . . stay only in the present. Watch your thoughts come and go. Don't try to ignore or suppress any thoughts and don't try to hold on to them. Simply *note* that they're there. Use your breathing to keep you anchored in the moment.

3. During your meditation it's normal for your attention to drift to stressful topics. Let this happen. And use a soft, tolerant, and accepting attitude toward any stressful thoughts and feelings that crop up. That is, just *observe* them. *Accept* that they're there. Let them just *exist* in your mind or body: a thought about something stressful, an unpleasant image, a physical sensation or pain. Stress comes from *reacting* to these mental and physical events, not from the events themselves. When you simply *notice* your thoughts and feelings without judgment, and return to focusing on your breathing (or your mantra), you'll be cultivating a mindful and less stressful relationship with them.

4. If you do find yourself responding to your thoughts and feelings—such as trying to push them out of your mind, exploring their logic, understanding where they're coming from, or catastrophizing and jumping to conclusions about them—switch back to simply *noticing* them and then return your attention to your breathing without getting caught up in the content of the thoughts.

5. Continue this process for as long as you'd like. When you're ready to stop, take a deep breath, exhale fully, and open your eyes. Say to yourself something like "I'm in the here and now."

Practicing mindfulness meditation trains you to be more in the present moment rather than suffering and focusing on the future or past. With enough practice, you'll be able to use this approach with stressful thoughts and feelings even when you're not meditating.

But mindfulness meditation is not an easy skill to learn. You must practice regularly if you want to benefit fully and truly become more mindful and accepting of the present. (You can also learn more about mindfulness with the help of some of the resources listed at the back of the book.) Practicing every day for 2 weeks, even if it's just for 10 minutes at a time, is a good start. As you feel more comfortable with the techniques, reduce your practice time to 20 to 30 minutes a few times per week. Keep track of your practicing using the Meditation Practice Log on page 189.

10

Maintaining a Healthy Lifestyle

Think about it: when you're starving, exhausted, stiff, and achy, you get grouchier and more irritable, your fuse is shorter, and you don't cope well with difficult situations. It's true for all of us. That's why healthy eating, physical fitness, and a good night's sleep are critical to managing stress. Of course the irony of maintaining a healthy lifestyle is that making changes in these daily routines can feel pretty stressful, especially if you know what you should be doing differently and you're inclined to beat yourself up for not doing it. So this chapter won't belabor the obvious, and its goal is certainly not to guilt you into adopting healthy habits. I'll give you proven, nonstressful ways to make any changes you decide might help, and I think you'll find some tricks and tips that you haven't heard before. Even small changes can make a big difference in reducing stress.

STRESS, NUTRITION, AND EATING

It's a vicious cycle: stress leads to unhealthy eating patterns, which lead to gaining weight, feeling lethargic, and maybe even guilty or depressed, which causes even more stress. How does it all start? For one thing, stress tempts you to eat the wrong foods—those high in sugar and fat—for comfort or to keep you distracted from your worries. We call this "emotional eating," and although these foods make you feel better in the moment, over time they make you pack on the pounds, especially if you're too stressed out to incorporate exercise and other activity into your lifestyle. The result is even more stress.

Emotional eating is using food to soothe stressful emotions like anger, sadness, worry, anxiety, guilt, boredom, and loneliness. It's triggered by major life events or daily hassles.

There's another way that stress leads to unhealthy eating: when you have lots to do and your day is full of hassles and deadlines, watching what you eat might be the last thing on your mind. As a result, you end up eating the easiest and most available foods—which are usually the least healthy. You might even skip meals, which leads to feeling hungry. And hunger clouds your judgment and makes you more impulsive, so you're more easily tempted by food that tastes good but isn't good for you. To make matters worse, high levels of cortisol, one of the stress hormones, cause the food you eat to be stored as fat, leading

Eating is a maladaptive way to deal with stress. Rather than turning to food, use the strategies in this workbook to help you manage stress and stressful emotions.

to more problems with weight control. The good news is that you can learn how to curb stress-related eating habits and develop healthy, stress-*reducing* patterns.

The Daily Food Diary

When you're stressed, your perception of what and how much you eat is often inaccurate. That's why keeping a food diary is the first step to successfully changing your eating habits. You can use the Daily Food Diary on the next page to help you keep track of what you eat and drink each day, what triggers you to eat, and how stressed out you feel when you eat. Make enough copies of the blank diary to last you for several weeks (or more) while you get comfortable with some shifts in eating. Here's how to fill it out:

Whether you create a binder or file, or just fold it up and put it in your pocket, keep your food diary (and a pencil) handy wherever you go so you can fill it out on the spot when you eat. If you wait very long, you'll forget the important information you need to include.

- **Date and time.** This will tell you when you tend to eat in ways that might be targets for change: Do you eat more on weekends than on weekdays? Do you tend to eat late at night?

- **Food.** Write down *everything* and be *specific*. Instead of writing "lunch," list everything that lunch includes: two hot dogs, two buns, ketchup, french fries, and a can of diet soda (see Maurice's sample Daily Food Diary on page 197). Don't forget about beverages, gum, candy, shakes, and other edibles not typically considered food. They might not be substantial, but they *do* count. Many of these foods, for example, contain lots of sugar.

Keeping track of whatever you eat makes you think more carefully about what you're putting in your mouth. It's a research-proven weight-loss strategy.

- **Amount and servings.** Here too, be specific: Don't enter just "doughnuts" but "3 doughnuts" if you want this diary to be revealing enough to help you control how much or what you eat. Use the nutrition labels on all packaged food to enter the

DAILY FOOD DIARY FOR _____
(day of the week and date of the year)

Time	Food	Amount/ # of servings	Place	Triggers	Stress level (0 to 10)

DAILY FOOD DIARY: MAURICE

Time	Food	Amount/ # of servings	Place	Triggers	Stress level
6:30 P.M.	Hamburgers	2	McDonald's	Dinnertime	4
	Fries	1 (large)		"	
	Regular Coke	1 large + refill		"	
	Sundae	1		"	
8:45	Pretzels	2 servings	TV room	Hunger	6
11:00	Ice cream (for a sundae)	2 servings	TV room	Hungry and bored	5
	Chocolate syrup	2 servings			

number of servings, whether it's "1 cup" of macaroni and cheese or "15" potato chips.

- **Place.** *Where* you eat matters, too. At home, for example, you're more likely to overeat when you're in front of the television because you're not paying attention to what's going into your mouth. And regularly eating out at restaurants contributes to weight gain because the portions tend to be large, cooked with fattening ingredients, and doused with calorie-rich sauces. Be specific: If you're out, write down where you're eating. If you're home, note which room of the house you're in.

- **Triggers.** You might eat for many reasons: you're feeling hungry, you're stressed, bored, you get a craving for a certain food, or you see an ad for something that looks good.

- **Stress level.** Keep track of your stress levels when you eat so you can recognize when you're falling victim to emotional eating.

Choosing the Best Foods for Reducing Stress

Food, just like medications, can cause psychological changes by changing levels of neurotransmitters and other chemicals in your brain and body. Food that contains lots of sugar, for example—like chocolate and other sweets—makes you feel euphoric because of the sudden increase in blood sugar levels. Choosing high-fiber unrefined carbohydrates over "quick" sugar can help you perform better under stress. There are numerous sources of information and advice on adopting a healthy diet (see the Resources for a few of the best) that you can tap to get more detail, but for optimal overall health and weight control, the following are some well-researched guidelines. Note that you can find out where a *packaged* food stands on nutrients such as sugar and fiber—and therefore whether it's likely to be a stress *inducer* or a stress *reducer*—simply by reading the nutrition label. Most experts today agree, however, that foods in their natural state—fresh fruits and vegetables (full of necessary vitamins and minerals), fresh protein like fish and meat, and whole grains—are the best way to go. For the nutrient content of these foods, it's a great help to have a book that lists nutrients for a wide variety of foods; again, see the Resources.

Serving Size

Pay attention to the amount listed as one serving (on a package label or in a nutrient count book)—it's often less than you're used to, and if you eat more than one serving, all the other nutrients you're consuming increase proportionately.

Calories, Fat, and Cholesterol

As a general rule, given the reality that we often eat more than one food at a time, 40 calories per serving size is fairly low, 100 calories per serving is moderate, and 400

Cutting Back on Alcohol

Back in Part I you learned why using alcohol is a maladaptive and potentially harmful way to handle stress (page 36). Alcohol also contains lots of calories but no healthy nutrients. Cutting back might be hard, but if you tend to drink in response to stress you'll want to try out these strategies:

1. **Switch to a drink with less alcohol or sugar.** Beers, wines, and mixed drinks vary widely in their alcohol content. Many cocktails contain mixes that are high in sugar. Look up what's in your favorite beverage and see if you can find a more healthy alternative.

2. **Drink double-fisted . . . your drink and a large glass of water.** Use the water to quench your thirst and sip the alcoholic drink for the flavor and enjoyment. The water will help you feel full and you'll have fewer alcoholic drinks.

3. **Let others know you're cutting back on your drinking.** This may stop them from urging you on.

4. **Meet friends at a coffee bar, not a tavern.** If the point of getting together is to hang out in a sociable environment, find a place where you won't be as tempted to drink too much alcohol. And if the plan is to watch a sporting event, have the party at someone's house rather than a sports bar.

5. **Keep track of how much money you spend on alcohol each week or month.** You might get sticker shock! But then, try to cut this amount in half. You'll save money along with calories.

EYE OPENER

Counting Carbs

A good way to follow a low-stress diet is to look at the discrepancy between the grams of total carbohydrates and grams of sugars per serving. Foods that have a big difference—meaning there are probably more *natural* than *added* sugars—are stress *reducers*. On the other hand, the closer the number of grams of sugar is to the total carbohydrates, the less healthy the food. **So, subtracting the grams of sugar from the grams of total carbohydrate is helpful in comparing the nutritional value of foods. Choose the food with the greatest discrepancy.**

calories or more is high—do your best to avoid foods with this many calories per serving. Also limit your calories from fat to about 30% of your total calories (the equivalent of 3 or fewer grams of fat for every 100 calories in a serving, since a gram of fat has 9 calories). For heart health, favor *unsaturated fats*, from nuts, fish, and olive oil, over *saturated* and *trans fats*, from animal products and hydrogenated oils (which are solid at room temperature, like vegetable shortening). Dietary cholesterol can increase the risk of heart disease in the same way that saturated fats do, so it's a good idea to keep your consumption of cholesterol down too.

Sodium and Potassium

If you're stressed out, try to limit your sodium intake to less than 2,400 mg per day since high levels are associated with high blood pressure and increased risk of stroke. It's smart to keep low-salt (or unsalted) chips, pretzels, and nuts in the house and to choose fresh meats, rather than cured meats such as bacon and salami. On the other hand, potassium is good for you. Your muscles and nerves need a healthy supply to function properly. Good sources of this nutrient include bananas, melons, potatoes, and low-fat milk.

Carbohydrates

The healthiest sources of carbohydrates are high-fiber foods like fruits and vegetables, whole-grain cereals, breads, pasta, and brown rice, which can keep you feeling full and help you avoid overeating. Check food labels and try to eat at least six servings of high-fiber foods per day.

Sugar

A stress-reducing diet should include no more than 40 grams of sugar per day. It can be an eye-opening experience to check sugar quantities on food labels—doing so might help you cut back on your sugar intake.

Protein

Proteins are your body's building blocks. They make sure your skin, muscles, brain, bones, blood vessels, and immune system are healthy and strong. As a rule of thumb, aim for between 50 and 75 grams of protein per day, preferably from beans and legumes, almonds, and lean meats (less than 3 grams of fat per serving) such as fish and poultry.

Modifying Your Diet the Low-Stress Way

After you've kept your food diary for a week, see which foods you tend to eat often and then look at their nutrient content. Doing so may immediately tell you where you'd like to make a few changes. But wait! Don't just go cold turkey (pardon the pun!) and make drastic changes all at once—they'll be hard to stick to and only stress you out more. You'll be much more successful if you make changes to your diet by going slowly and gradually:

EYE PENER

Eating Out

Dining in social situations and restaurants presents special challenges for trying to maintain healthy eating habits. You're at higher risk of overeating because of the large portion sizes, and you're likely to consume foods high in calories from fat and sugar because of how food is cooked when you're out. Here are some things you can do to stay as healthy as possible:

- Plan ahead. When you know you're going to be at a party or restaurant later in the day, adjust your other meals to be lighter and healthier.

- Choose broiled, baked, or grilled selections, which are healthier than their fried counterparts.

- Ask for sauces and dressings on the side so you can control how much of these high-fat toppings you eat.

- Share a dessert with someone or order fruit, low-fat yogurt, or fruit sherbet.

- Drink lots of water to keep you feeling full.

- Don't clean your plate. Most portions at restaurants are extremely large. When you receive your meal, decide what you'll eat and what you'll leave. If you really like the food, take your leftovers home.

- If you eat lunch at work, bring your own from home rather than going to a restaurant.

- Avoid buffets if you can; but if not, go through the line once and get a salad while you look at what else is there. Then, while you're eating your salad, plan the rest of your meal. Use another salad plate when you go through the line again and you'll automatically eat less.

DIETARY CHANGES I WANT TO TRY TO REDUCE STRESS

Stress-*producing* foods I want to cut back on: _____

_____

_____

Stress-*reducing* foods I want to try to eat more of: _____

_____

_____

I can replace _____ with _____

I can replace _____ with _____

I can replace _____ with _____

I can replace _____ with _____

- If you drink five cans of soda each day, try cutting back to four cans for a week or two, then to three cans, and so on until you're within the recommended daily sugar levels.

- If you eat a bowl of sugary cereal every morning for breakfast, try *half* a bowl and a piece of whole-wheat toast.

- If you don't eat any fruits or vegetables, start by adding a single serving somewhere in your day. After a week, add another serving.

In the worksheet above, plan how you can gradually make stress-busting changes to your eating over the next few weeks or months. You might plan to cut back on foods that cause stress, substitute stress-reducing choices for stress-inducing foods, or add more stress–reducing foods.

Defeating Overeating

Overeating leads to stress because it makes you feel full and lethargic, and it contributes to weight gain. Unfortunately, the goal of controlling your consumption can seem overwhelming—just another thing to pay attention to when your "plate" is already full. Here are some low-stress ways to take steps in the right direction:

- **Serve and eat one helping of food at a time.** If you want two slices of toast, make one and eat it before making the second. If you want two pieces of meat loaf, put one on your plate and finish it before going back for more. Maybe you'll pass up the extra serving(s).

- **Keep serving plates away from the table.** Leave the pan on the stove or the platter in a different room. Don't eat directly from bags of chips or boxes of cookies; take one serving at a time. This won't keep you from having seconds, but it interrupts the process of overeating.

- **Slow down and try to make your meals last as long as possible.** If you're stressed and constantly on the go, you probably eat too *fast*. It takes about 20 minutes from the time you start eating for your brain to let you know that your stomach's full. Therefore, when you eat quickly, you don't realize you're full until you've had too much. If you take smaller bites, put your fork down after each bite, and take a sip of your beverage between bites, you'll feel full after having eaten less food. Try eating slowly and mindfully (see Chapter 9)—savoring every bite of food. Take a clock to the table and try to make your meals last at least 20 minutes. Wait for at least 5 minutes between helpings. This will slow your eating and give you more time to decide if you're really still hungry.

Use the log below to keep track of change strategies you try (make extra copies of the form). To keep the process low-stress, try out only one or two at a time for at least

DIETARY CHANGE LOG

Strategy	Date started	Notes and remarks
Serve one helping at a time		
Serving dishes away from table		
Don't eat directly from bag/box		
Small bites of food		
Put fork down between bites		
Take drink between bites		
Have meal last 20 minutes (clock)		
Wait 5 minutes between helpings		

EYE PENER

Eat *More*, Weigh *Less*, and Be Less Stressed

How many meals do you eat each day? If you're like most people, it's two or three large ones. But creating an eating schedule that includes smaller, more frequent "mini-meals" through the day helps you control your weight and be less stressed. That's because your body and mind run best when your blood sugar levels are stable—not too high, not too low. When you eat large meals, your blood sugar spikes and then *plunges*. It's this instability that leads to hunger and causes cravings for unhealthy foods and snacks between meals. The best way to keep your blood sugar stable is to eat four to six small but healthy meals throughout the day. Try high-protein foods such as nuts, eggs, lean meats, and cheese, and high-fiber foods such as fruits, vegetables, and whole grains. You'll digest your food more slowly, feel full for a longer time, and avoid hunger pangs (and cravings) between meals. Here's a sample daily "mini-meal" menu:

Breakfast (7:00 A.M.): Turkey and cheese omelet with a piece of whole-wheat toast or a serving of high-fiber cereal with fruit

Midmorning snack (10:00 A.M.): Handful of almonds and a cup of low-fat yogurt

Lunch (noon): Lean turkey on whole-wheat bread with lettuce, tomato, and mustard

Early afternoon snack (2:00P.M.): Choose from low-fat cheese (such as a mozzarella cheese stick), grapes or other berries, or peanut butter on whole-wheat toast

Late afternoon snack (4:00 P.M.): Something from the early afternoon snack list

Dinner and dessert (6:00 P.M.): Lean meat (such as a serving of chicken breast), salad, a vegetable; and for dessert, a serving of dark chocolate or low-fat ice cream. This meal is designed to keep you feeling full so you're less likely to have late-night feeding frenzies. You're highly prone to overindulge in unhealthy foods when you raid the kitchen at any point after dinner.

Now it's your turn: create your own "mini-meal" schedule below. What foods will you eat throughout the day?

Breakfast: Time _____ Foods: _____

Midmorning snack: Time _____ Foods: _____

Lunch: Time _____ Foods: _____

Early afternoon snack: Time _____ Foods: _____

Late afternoon snack: Time _____ Foods: _____

Dinner and dessert: Time _____ Foods: _____

EYE 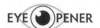 PENER

Breakfast: The Most Important Meal of the Day for Managing Stress

When you're under stress, it's easy to feel too busy to have breakfast. And if you're trying to lose weight, skipping meals might seem like a good idea too. But it's not. If you're going to successfully manage each day's stressors, you need to refuel your body each morning. Studies clearly show that eating breakfast improves your physical and mental abilities. What's more, it keeps you from feeling hungry so you're less likely to snack on unhealthy foods or overeat later on. So, whether it's to help you perform at your best, deal with that situation that's got you stressed out, or drop some weight, breakfast really is the most important meal of the day.

a week to get comfortable with your new patterns. Once these become second nature, make a few more changes, and so on.

Crushing your Cravings

Answer the following questions about your eating patterns by circling Yes or No:

1. Driving past a fast-food restaurant makes me want to eat.   Yes   No

2. When someone mentions a food I love, I feel like eating.   Yes   No

3. If I see something tasty sitting out, I can't resist eating—
   even if I just had a meal.   Yes   No

4. Even after eating a large meal, I still want dessert.   Yes   No

5. When I see a TV commercial for something delicious, I
   want to eat.   Yes   No

If you answered yes to some of these, it means you tend to eat in response to cravings (as opposed to actual hunger). This is very common when you're stressed out—but it's also unhealthy since you're likely to crave foods that cause stress: fatty, sugary, salty, and other unhealthy snacks (after all, they taste good and make you feel good). Here are some tips for successfully getting past cravings.

Cravings versus Real Hunger: Recognize the Difference

The first step to curbing your cravings is to learn the differences between genuine hunger (which is physical) and cravings (which are purely mental). You're probably familiar with the signs of real hunger: a rumbling stomach, irritability, headache, dizziness, and difficulty concentrating. Think of it this way: when you're hungry, your body is begging you for food. And it's important to eat when you notice hunger signs; otherwise you become ravenous and make impulsive (and usually poor) food choices.

A craving, on the other hand, is an intense emotional *desire* to eat a specific food. Whether you're hungry or full doesn't really matter. For example, you might have just finished eating a large meal—and feel full—but you still want that piece of cake you've been thinking about for dessert.

The Apple Test

Still can't tell if it's real hunger or just a craving? Try the *apple test*: Would an apple satisfy your hunger, or do you absolutely have to have the gooey brownie you just saw on TV? If it's genuine hunger, chances are you'll go with the apple.

Distract Yourself

If your "hunger" is really just a craving, get involved in an activity (besides eating) that will distract you and keep you engaged (preferably something that involves using your hands). But stay away from the kitchen (or wherever the food you crave is)! Here are some suggestions: Play computer games, give yourself a manicure/pedicure, knit or sew, exercise (jump rope, go for a walk, go to the gym, use a Wii Fit), play with your children or pet, enjoy some romantic time with your partner, or send e-mails. Tell yourself you've got to continue with your activity for 30 minutes before you satisfy the craving. Chances are the craving will have petered out when the time is up. In the following spaces, write down five activities you can do to distract yourself from food cravings:

1. _____   4. _____

2. _____   5. _____

3. _____

Fake Out Your Craving with Anti-Stress Foods

Rather than reaching for the ice cream or bag of chips, trick your craving by eating foods that contain a small amount of calories or carbohydrates but that are high in fiber, which digests slowly and makes you feel full. These anti-stress/anti-craving foods include almonds and other nuts; apples, bananas, and other fruits; raspberries and other berries; whole-grain cereal; popcorn; low-fat yogurt; a small amount of dark chocolate; and leafy green vegetables. An 8-ounce glass of water can also do the trick.

Indulge Once in a While

Finally, it's not the end of the world to give in to cravings once in a while. In fact, I recommend planning one meal per week when you'll satisfy your cravings and treat yourself to your favorite unhealthy foods. If you do this *once a week*, it won't hurt you and may even reduce your stress about having to resist giving in to your cravings. And after you indulge, your cravings may be less noticeable for a few days.

EXERCISE

Exercise is one of the best things you can do to relieve stress. It has both short- and long-term positive effects, including helping you get (or stay) physically fit, releasing tension, and helping you sleep better (see the section on sleep later in this chapter). Exercise also improves blood flow to your brain, which increases nutrients and helps to carry away waste products that build up when you're stressed. And you're probably aware that exercise increases levels of endorphins—chemicals that naturally create a sense of well-being. It's also true that as a result of exercise, your body's physical response to stress becomes less extreme. This means that exercising protects you against the severe physical and psychological effects of long-term stress.

Exercise can be divided into *programmed* and *lifestyle* exercise. Programmed exercise involves taking time out of your normal daily routine specifically for the purpose of exercise. Lifestyle exercise is exercise that you incorporate as part of your normal routine. I'll help you include both in your stress management repertoire.

Planning an Exercise Program

Let's get the hard part out of the way right now: If exercising isn't already part of your routine, making time for it can be a challenge. After all, you're too busy enough as it is, right? Do you even have the time to exercise? Before you decide that you don't, consider that the time you invest in exercising will pay huge dividends down the road—you've read about its beneficial effects. Exercising is a stress reducer. After you get out there you'll not only feel better physically, but you'll be sharper mentally and ready to return to work, parenting, or whatever is next on your agenda.

So, let's consider some logistics: Can you adjust your morning schedule, such as waking up earlier to exercise? Can you exercise during your break at work? Can you find someone to watch the kids while you walk or bike?

To make exercising more enjoyable, go with a friend or family member. This can also keep you motivated and sticking to your schedule. Or, if you're by yourself, take music with you and listen using headphones. You might need to give it a few weeks, but once you settle into a routine, you'll begin to notice the mental and physical benefits of exercising; and you'll look forward to your exercise sessions. You might even decide to join a fitness center or hire a personal trainer to help you expand your exercising habits. Consider how you'll make the time to exercise, and how you can make it enjoyable. Write down your plans in the following spaces:

What days of the week will I exercise? _____

What time of day is best for me to exercise? _____

Whom will I exercise with? _____

If alone, what music will I listen to? _____

How else can I make exercise more enjoyable? _____

Barriers to Exercising

Sticking to an exercise routine isn't easy—there are plenty of potential obstacles: time, boredom, injuries, self-confidence, to name a few. But these don't need to stand in your way. Use the worksheet below to identify the possible barriers to success with *your* exercise program. Then generate solutions to each challenge. You might use what you learned about problem solving in Chapter 5 to help you.

Choosing an Exercise

The exercises that reduce stress most are those that require the use of large muscle groups and use up lots of energy. Walking and biking are excellent examples. Slower-

PROBLEM-SOLVING OBSTACLES TO EXERCISING

Barriers to exercising	Solutions

paced exercises, such as stretching, are not as useful because you're not expending much energy. If you don't exercise regularly, I recommend walking as your primary form of programmed exercise. You can walk alone or with others, at any time of the day, indoors or outdoors, at home, at work, or on vacation; and it doesn't require any special equipment. Riding a bicycle (regular or stationary) can be a good alternative to walking. If you already exercise regularly, you might skip to the section on lifestyle exercise. In the following blank, write down the exercise(s) you'll do as part of your stress management program.

What exercise(s) will I do? _____

Setting Goals and Tracking Progress

There are different ways you can set goals for exercising. One way is to set a *time* goal, such as walking for 20 minutes on each of 3 days a week. Another strategy is to set a *distance* goal, such as walking half a mile 3 days a week. If you don't exercise regularly, begin with easier goals and increase them each week; for example, walking for 10 minutes 4 days a week during the first week of your program, 15 minutes 4 days during the second week, and 20 minutes on each of 4 days during the third week. I recommend walking at a leisurely pace and using time goals at first, since it's the easiest to measure. Later on, you could switch to distance goals if you want to increase your walking speed. Finally, I suggest warming up with a few minutes of stretching before each exercise session. This reduces the chances of straining any muscles. Write your goals on a copy of the Programmed Exercise Record Form on the next page. Here's a set of sample goals for beginning an exercising (walking) program:

Sample Weekly Goals for a Walking Program

Week 1: Walk for 15 minutes on 3 days

Week 2: Walk for 20 minutes on 3 days

Week 3: Walk for 30 minutes on 3 days

Week 4: Walk for 40 minutes on 3 days

Week 5: Walk for 50 minutes on 3 days

Now start using the Programmed Exercise Record Form as a calendar on which you keep track of the number of minutes you spend exercising each day. You've set a goal for each week. So, at the end of the week, determine whether you've met this goal. Make as many copies of the blank form as you think you'll need (one per month) until exercising becomes part of your regular routine.

PROGRAMMED EXERCISE RECORD FORM

Month: _____

	Week 1	Week 2	Week 3	Week 4	Week 5
Goal for the week					
Monday					
Tuesday					
Wednesday					
Thursday					
Friday					
Saturday					
Sunday					
Goal achieved?					

From *The Stress Less Workbook*. Copyright 2012 by The Guilford Press.

Incorporating Exercise into Your Daily Life

Rather than walking down the hall to talk to a coworker, do you stay at your desk and send an e-mail? Do you take the elevator instead of the stairs? Do you keep searching for that perfect parking spot near the mall or store, rather than parking farther away and walking? Do you spend all day in stressful meetings only to come home and lounge in front of the TV? When you're overwhelmed with stress, it's easy to drift into a sedentary lifestyle in which your daily level of physical activity dwindles. But with a little creativity and planning, you can make small changes to include more lifestyle exercise and help reduce stress. Your mindset should be this: *How can I take advantage of opportunities to use my muscles more?* On the next page are some ideas:

- Take the stairs instead of the elevator.

- Walk rather than drive. If you have to drive, park a little father from your destination and walk the rest of the way.

- Take exercise breaks during the day—get up, walk around, stretch, and relax.

- Consciously reduce how much you rely on motorized machines. For example, mow your lawn with a push mower instead of a riding mower. Rake the leaves and shovel the snow instead of using a leaf or snow blower.

- The next time you mail a letter, walk to the mailbox on the *next* block.

- Stand while you work, if possible. Or buy a stability (exercise) ball and sit on it rather than on your chair.

- Substitute active behaviors (such as bowling, hiking, or dancing) for sedentary ones (such as computer games, TV, or movies) whenever possible.

Take advantage of at least one opportunity each day to increase your lifestyle exercise. On the first day, for instance, walk an extra flight of stairs instead of taking the elevator all the way up. On the second day, park at the *far* end of the parking lot at work, or on the next block, if you're visiting a friend. In the worksheet below, write your plan for increasing lifestyle exercise this week.

SLEEPING WELL

You're probably all too familiar with how sleep (and the lack of it) can affect your stress level. After a good night's sleep, you feel refreshed and more positive about facing the

---

MY ONE-WEEK PLAN FOR INCREASING LIFESTYLE EXERCISE

Day 1: _____

Day 2: _____

Day 3: _____

Day 4: _____

Day 5: _____

Day 6: _____

Day 7: _____

day. On the other hand, after a sleepless night (or maybe several of them in a row), you're more irritable, short-tempered, and more easily thrown into bouts of anxiety or depression—the perfect recipe for a stress-filled day. Lack of sleep also saps other stress management essentials, such as your energy level and your ability to think clearly and concentrate.

And it's a vicious cycle. Being stressed leads back to more sleep problems. Remember that stress is a state of heightened alertness and arousal, which is actually the *opposite* of how your body needs to feel for you to enjoy a good night's sleep. And when you stay up late at night to work or worry about stressors, you throw your sleep schedule out of balance, further confusing your body. Do you use caffeine to help you stay awake, or alcohol and tobacco products to help you relax? These also affect how you sleep. Luckily, there are effective strategies to help you break the vicious cycle between stress and poor sleep. You'll learn how to use them in this section.

Sleep Hygiene

Your *sleep hygiene* is your bedtime behavior—in other words, your own set of habits that determine how well you sleep. Most people who sleep well develop lifestyle patterns that promote sound sleep (including eating healthy and exercising). But stress interrupts all that, leading to poor sleep hygiene. Problematic bedtime habits can also come from not knowing how to set up your sleeping environment and prepare for going to bed, or what to do when you can't get to sleep. Let's start with some questions to assess your own sleep hygiene. Fill out the worksheet on the next page to get an idea of the quality of your sleep hygiene.

This is one of those tests where a higher score means you've probably got more to work on. If you don't feel like you get enough sound sleep (see the Eye Opener on the next page) and you circled lots of 1's and 2's, your sleep hygiene could use an upgrade. Read this section carefully and try out the recommendations. On the other hand, if you've circled mainly 0's and you're someone who sleeps soundly, you might skip this part of the chapter.

Optimizing Your Sleep Environment

Your surroundings have a lot to do with how well you sleep. And while some people can easily adjust to changes in their sleep environment, when you're stressed it's more difficult. All the more reason to make sure your sleep environment is optimal. Here are some recommendations:

Make sure you feel comfortable in your bed and with your pillow. Everyone's different, but if your sleeping place isn't cozy and pleasant, how can you expect to fully relax? A visit to a mattress store might be worthwhile, even if it requires a financial outlay. You can't put a price on a good night's sleep.

Also, make sure your room is dark and quiet. If too much light is getting in, try heavier curtains or shutters, or change the lighting outside your room or house. For

MY SLEEP HYGIENE

Circle the most appropriate number.

0 = Never   1 = Sometimes   2 = Always

1. I exercise within a few hours of going to bed.	0	1	2
2. I finish my last full meal of the day within two hours of bedtime.	0	1	2
3. I do work in bed when I can't sleep.	0	1	2
4. I go to sleep at different times each night.	0	1	2
5. I worry about (or have intense discussions about) problems in bed.	0	1	2
6. My bedroom is lit up, even at night when I'm trying to sleep.	0	1	2
7. I try to go to bed when I'm not really tired.	0	1	2
8. I have alcoholic or caffeinated drinks within a few hours of bedtime.	0	1	2
9. I spend a lot of "awake time" in bed (or in the bedroom).	0	1	2
10. I keep my bedroom warm, and I sweat when I sleep.	0	1	2

EYE 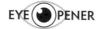 OPENER

How Much Sleep Do I Need?

Disregard what you've heard—there's no one-size-fits-all answer to this question since everyone's sleep needs are a little different. But there are ways to tell if you're not getting enough sleep. Here they are:

- **The alarm clock test:** If you need an alarm to wake you up, you're not getting enough sleep. Try going to bed 15 minutes earlier. Do you still need an alarm clock? If you do, push your bedtime up another 15 minutes. Keep adding 15 minutes until you no longer need the alarm to wake you up. This should give you a pretty good idea of the amount of sleep you need per night.

- **The nap test:** Do you get tired and need a "power nap" during the day? If so, you're not getting enough sleep at night. Try going to bed 30 to 60 minutes earlier.

- **The caffeine test:** How much coffee do you drink? If you're drinking caffeinated beverages to stay awake, you're probably not getting enough sleep.

example, turn off the hall light or point the spotlights in a different direction outside. Loud, irregular, or unpredictable noise also hampers your sleep. If the noise is coming from outside, close your windows, use heavy curtains, and consider installing carpet and bookshelves (and other wall hangings) to absorb some of the unwanted noise. Alternatively, you can use a more acceptable sound—such as white noise—to mask the undesirable ones. White noise is "background noise" such as the sound of a waterfall, crickets chirping, the beach, or even the constant hum of an air conditioner on a summer night. Some smartphones and alarm clocks will play white noise, or you can buy a sound generator or CD with white noise tracks that you can play as you're going to bed. When all else fails, you might try earplugs.

Believe it or not, the temperature of your bedroom can also affect how you sleep. That's because when you go to sleep, your body lowers its temperature a bit, and if the room is too hot or too cold, your body has to work harder to make this happen—which interrupts sleep. Because the drop in body temperature actually helps put you to sleep, you'll sleep better in a cooler room than in a warmer one. But if it's too cold or too hot, you're less likely to sleep well. Experts agree that a room temperature of between 65 and 72 degrees Fahrenheit is ideal, but everyone's a little different, so you need to find your ideal sleeping temperature. Cold feet can be especially disruptive to sleep, so you might try wearing socks to bed.

> *Think of your bedroom as a cave. It should be cool, quiet, and dark.*

What to Do and Not Do *before* Bed

Just like an athlete goes through a pregame ritual to get him- or herself "in the zone" and ready for competition, you'll sleep better if you have a pre-bedtime routine that sets the stage for settling down for the day. Here's what your routine should (and shouldn't) include:

- **Get on schedule.** We all have an internal ("circadian") clock that controls our sleep–wake cycle. When we get into a pattern of going to sleep (and waking up) at about the same time each day, it strengthens this clock and helps you fall asleep faster, sleep more deeply, and wake up more easily. Try scheduling a time to stop working and to begin unwinding to prepare for bedtime.

- **Take a bath.** Remember when you were a child and you took a bath at the end of the day before going to sleep? You're older now, but a warm, relaxing bath will still have the same soothing effect. This is an excellent way to separate the daily worries and hassles from sleep time.

- **Do something relaxing.** Read a chapter of a book. Listen to some mellow music, meditate, or use relaxation strategies (see Chapter 9) before you call it a night. If you have a bed partner, ask for a massage. Do whatever allows your brain to separate the hassles of the day from sleep time.

- **Watch what you eat.** Although it's not essential, a light (healthy) snack before bed can't hurt. In fact, eating foods that contain tryptophan—a substance that induces sleep—can help you get to sleep easier. Try low-fat dairy products such as milk and cheese.

  On the other hand, make sure to avoid heavy meals within a few hours of bedtime. When your stomach is very full, you might feel uncomfortable or have indigestion, which will keep you from settling down into sleep. And watch what you eat in the evenings as well. Spicy foods can cause heartburn, gas, or bloating, which leads to difficulty falling asleep and discomfort during the night. To cut down on overnight trips to the bathroom, try restricting fluids close to bedtime.

- **Don't exercise too close to bedtime.** Getting regular exercise helps you sleep better and longer—but not if you exercise right before going to bed. You'll actually have a harder time falling asleep since, in addition to making you more alert, exercising raises your body temperature for as much as 6 hours (remember, cooler is better for good sleep). Although you already have a hectic schedule, try to get your workout in early in the morning or in the late afternoon/early evening (before eating dinner).

- **Avoid stimulants.** Caffeine and nicotine are stimulants that increase your heart rate and muscle tension and excite your brain. Although moderate daytime use of caffeine probably won't hamper your sleep at night, having tea, coffee, soda, or chocolate close to bedtime causes sleep problems. Similarly, if you're a smoker, don't smoke before bed. There's good news, though—smokers who quit their habit often sleep much better once the withdrawal effects of nicotine subside.

- **Don't overdo the alcohol.** Alcohol slows the brain's activity; and although this might help you get to sleep at first, when you drink large quantities of alcohol, you're more likely to have trouble with awakening in the middle of the night and not being able to fall back to sleep. You might also experience the classic "hangover" effects such as nausea, dizziness, and headaches, which will keep you from enjoying a restful sleep.

What to Do and Not Do *in* Bed

Humans make associations between things all the time. For example, no doubt you've learned to associate the color green with "go" or "start" and red with "stop." Maybe you associate certain songs with particular memories, thoughts, and feelings. Feeling sleepy can also become associated with certain situations. For some people, just sitting on the couch can trigger drowsiness. This might occur if the person repeatedly naps on that particular couch. In other words, feeling drowsy and napping become associated with the couch because they're repeatedly paired together—a process called "classical conditioning." For people who sleep well, feeling drowsy when they get into bed has become a conditioned response because these two things (being in bed and going to sleep) are paired together on a nightly basis . . . and that's a good thing.

But if you have trouble sleeping, being in bed has probably become paired with feeling awake and with anxiety and stress over your unsuccessful attempts to get to sleep. In fact, you might have negative thoughts and feelings that are triggered by the whole process of getting ready for bed each night. And this will make falling asleep extremely difficult (imagine trying to adjust if green suddenly meant "stop" and red meant "go"!). If you end up sleeping on the couch or a chair because you're no longer able to fall asleep in the bedroom, this is probably what's going on. Luckily, though, with practice you can reestablish the connection between bedtime, your bed, and rapidly falling asleep. The main idea is to decrease how much awake time you spend when you're in bed. Here are some tips.

- **Go to bed only when you're drowsy.** Remember that being *drowsy* isn't the same as being *tired*. The signs of drowsiness include drooping eyelids, a nodding head, and yawning. This will help prevent you from spending time lying in bed having negative thoughts about sleep—thoughts about how bad it will be if you don't get enough sleep and about everything you have to do in the morning. These just create more stress and make it harder to fall asleep.

- **Use the 20-minute rule.** If you don't fall asleep after about 20 minutes, get up and go to another room to do something relaxing—maybe some light reading or a relaxation technique—until you do feel drowsy again. Then go back to bed and repeat this as often as necessary until you fall asleep. Don't do anything too stimulating, like work or watch horror movies. This will only increase your arousal level and make it harder to fall asleep.

- **Don't watch the clock.** Counting the minutes when you can't fall asleep will only create more stress since you're bound to catastrophize about how much sleep you're missing and how terrible you'll feel in the morning. For example, thoughts like "If I don't get to sleep soon, I won't be able to function at all tomorrow" all but guarantee that you'll have trouble falling asleep. If you find yourself having these kinds of thoughts, try the techniques in Chapter 8 for managing stress-related thoughts. If you find yourself watching the clock in bed, turn it so it's facing the other way.

- **Use your bed only for sleep and sexual activity.** Don't do things in bed that are incompatible with sleeping. For example, avoid eating, watching TV (especially political shows on cable that are designed to provoke your ire at the other party), studying for that big final exam, or working on your IRS tax audit. These are bound to arouse you and make it difficult to fall asleep. Repeatedly engaging in these kinds of activities helps condition arousal to the bed environment when instead you want to condition a feeling of relaxation to being in bed.

Part III

Making Stress Management Techniques Work in Your Daily Life

11

Managing Stress at Work

Ask most people in the workforce and they'll tell you that their job ranks among their greatest sources of stress. It's not easy trying to be "on" every day and knowing that you're under the boss's lens whenever you're "off." And even if your performance is pretty stellar most of the time, your job security is subject to countless other factors outside your control. For one thing, layoffs and budget cuts affect everyone either directly or indirectly, and the result is increased fear, uncertainty, and higher levels of stress since you're forced to do more with less. Since job stress grows in rough economic times, it's important to learn ways of coping with the pressure. But work causes stress in deeper, more personal ways too. Often our self-image is tied up with how much we succeed and get ahead. Maybe you set standards and then compete with yourself to meet or surpass them. How much does it bruise your ego when you're passed over for a promotion or award? And to top it off, no matter how talented you are, your success depends a lot on your relationships with other people—employers, coworkers, bosses, and the like. Not only does this add another layer of stress; it can also complicate how you manage your stress.

Your Own Work Stress

To start with, let's figure out the causes of your own work stress. Some of your stressors might be easy to identify. Do you work long hours? Does your boss ride you hard or act inconsiderate? Maybe you've got a personality clash with a coworker or you're feeling at risk of being laid off.

Don't overlook more subtle stressors either. Do you beat yourself up when you don't close every deal or your numbers drop a fraction or someone else comes up with an idea you "should" have thought of first? Are you feeling lousy about an important project or performance review that didn't go as well as expected? Perhaps the general climate of your workplace is extremely tense or hectic.

Finally, could there be underlying personal factors that affect your levels of work stress? For instance, do you have problems speaking in front of other people? Do you feel like you disappear into the woodwork when the plum assignments or awards are handed out because you don't like to put yourself forward? Do you anger easily and inadvertently alienate coworkers? Do you overwork yourself or demand perfection? Are you someone who doesn't do well with making changes? Do you need constant reassurance or positive feedback? Is your own sense of self-worth closely tied to how things are going at work? Recognizing these vulnerabilities will help you head off potential problems before they cause too much stress.

Consider what's stressing you out about work and then list your most stressful events, situations, feelings, and personal vulnerabilities in the worksheet at the bottom of the page. If you're having a hard time pinpointing them, use the My Problem Cues worksheet from Chapter 5 (page 86) to help you.

Fortunately, there are lots of things you can do to reduce the stress you feel on the job. In this chapter, I'll cover some particularly stressful situations you might encounter at work and show you how to tailor the techniques you learned in Part II to help you manage them.

NOT ENOUGH PERSONAL TIME

Right off the bat, one thing that's almost certain to be a source of stress is not having enough "me time" to relax, enjoy a good movie or book, or even take proper care of yourself. As you learned in Chapter 10, eating healthily, exercising, and getting a good night's rest are critical to staying at the top of your game and fighting stress—at work too. But maybe the pressure is so great, and the hours so long, that you've put your own health on the back burner. If that's the case, it's worth using the time management strategies in Chapter 7 to help you prioritize.

Shari was an elementary school teacher who was truly dedicated to her students.

MY SOURCES OF WORK STRESS

1. _____

2. _____

3. _____

4. _____

5. _____

6. _____

7. _____

From the moment she woke up to the time her head hit the pillow at night, she was either teaching or thinking about teaching—formulating lesson plans, grading papers, communicating with parents, and the like. But family and leisure time, not to mention her health, had gone by the wayside. She'd ignored not-so-subtle pleas from her husband and kids to "leave work at work," and she'd avoided hopping on the scale to see how much weight she'd gained since her clothes were feeling tighter and tighter. But it was when she started consistently feeling sleepy in the middle of the day that she put the time management exercises in Chapter 7 to work. These helped Shari examine more carefully how she was spending her time, revisit her priorities, and decide on some changes. She reduced a number of low-priority activities, mostly by delegating them to her teacher's aide, and she started saying "no" more often when asked to organize events at school. As a result, she was able to spend more quality time with her family without feeling guilty, get daily exercise (by taking long walks during her lunch break), find time to read recipes and cook healthy meals, and get to bed earlier to ensure a good night's sleep. If you feel like your workday never ends and you're starting to feel stressed out by never getting away from the job, go back to Chapter 7 and take a close, hard look at how you can divide up your time differently.

DEALING WITH A DIFFICULT BOSS OR TEACHER

Meet Mike, who works in the marketing department of a publishing company. He'd been there for a few months when his boss quit and was replaced by Nick, who knew a lot about selling books but wasn't very good at managing people. Within a few weeks of having Nick as his new boss, Mike was hating every hour on the job, and after suffering through each day, he blew up when he got home, yelling first at his wife and then at the kids, before grabbing a beer and flopping down in front of the TV. Sleep brought him no rest, and he couldn't let go of his tension over the weekend, making it a challenge for anyone to be around him. This made it doubly hard for Mike to feel like his normal self.

According to Mike, Nick changed deadlines without telling Mike and then humiliated him in front of coworkers for not getting his work done on time. He also stole some of Mike's best ideas, passing them off as his own in staff meetings. Nick piled on the work too, so Mike felt obligated to stay at the office late, take work home, and come in so early he never saw his family in the morning—to say nothing of being unavailable to help his wife with the kids and household. And, Mike declared, it was all personal, as evidenced by Nick's snide comments like "Hey, Mike, you must have just stepped out of a time machine if you're still wearing clothes like that!" What could Mike do? He wanted to quit his job, but he couldn't—not in this economy—so he was trapped.

Put yourself in Mike's shoes. What would make him less stressed? A better relationship with Nick? More respect and recognition at work? Maybe he'd be satisfied with a reduction in his workload. Perhaps cultivating a relationship with a coworker—someone to blow off steam with—would help. Would it help to analyze and change the way he thinks about any of this? What would help *you* feel less stressed in a situation like this?

What should Mike's next step be? Is there really no way out of this stress? Following are the stress management techniques you learned about in Part II. On the line to the left of each technique, prioritize how you'd suggest Mike address his work stress by ranking the techniques first, second, third, and so on (you don't have to use *all* of them). Then, on the line to the right of each technique, briefly describe your plan for using this strategy. How can he use the strategies to reduce his stress? The priority list and plans that Mike came up with himself follow.

_____ Problem solving: _____

_____

_____ Communication/assertiveness: _____

_____

_____ Time management: _____

_____

_____ Cognitive therapy: _____

_____

_____ Muscle relaxation: _____

_____

_____ Meditation: _____

_____

_____ Healthy lifestyle: _____

_____

Mike's Priority List and Plan for Managing His Work Stress

___1___ Problem solving: *Go and talk directly with Nick about their relationship*

_____

___2___ Communication/assertiveness: *Stand up for myself, but make sure not to*
offend Nick; develop more relationships with coworkers; ask for reduced workload

___7___ Time management: *Might make the workload seem a bit less*

_____

___3___ Cognitive therapy: *Change how I think when a situation can't be changed*

_____

___5___ Muscle relaxation: *After a confrontation, I can relax, but will it solve my*
problems?

___6___ Meditation: _____*This can help me ease my mind, but it won't solve my*_____

_____*problems with Nick*_____

___4___ Healthy lifestyle: ___*Go back to stopping at the gym on the way home, even if*___

_____*it means leaving some work undone to make the time*___

As you can see, Mike decided to start with problem solving. His wife, eager to have her husband involved with his family again, suggested Mike just march into Nick's office and say that he was not going to put up with this treatment anymore. While Mike knew assertive communication was probably going to be necessary with Nick, he was so exhausted from stress and overwork that he couldn't muster the energy and conviction to lay down the law with anyone, even the family dog. So he took the step-by-step problem-solving approach first.

Mike scheduled a time to meet individually with Nick, but thinking about what he'd say made his anxiety soar. The only way he found to stay focused on his goal was to go back to Chapter 6 and remind himself of the guidelines for assertiveness. He also used the tips in the Eye Opener on page 225.

What happened in the meeting? Mike was assertive (in his demeanor, his words, and his body language). Without making accusations, he let Nick know that he wasn't happy with their relationship and hoped to smooth things over. He was specific about what he didn't like (being scolded in front of coworkers, having his ideas stolen, and feeling overworked) and what he'd prefer (discussing problems in private, getting greater recognition for his work, and having a more manageable workload). In response, Nick was reasonable. He listened to Mike, and the two even hammered out a plan for reducing Mike's workload. Although they didn't really get around to addressing the relationship or recognition issues, Mike felt that he had gotten somewhere; and in the end he told Nick he appreciated the chance to meet and discuss these issues.

And things were better—at least for a while. Mike's workload was more manageable and things were better at home. He felt more himself, slept better at night, and was more pleasant to be around. After a few weeks, though, Nick was back at it again. There were snide comments, bullying, and criticism in front of coworkers, and Mike even found out that Nick had passed around and represented as his own a publicity plan that Mike had

---

The Five Steps to Effective Problem Solving

Step 1: Recognizing problems

Step 2: Choosing and clarifying a problem to solve

Step 3: Brainstorming solutions

Step 4: Narrowing down the possibilities

Step 5: Developing and carrying out an action plan

THE FIVE STEPS TO EFFECTIVE PROBLEM SOLVING: MIKE

Step 1: Recognizing problems—*(1) I feel overwhelmed by my workload. (2) Nick keeps taking credit for my ideas. (3) Nick constantly makes snide and embarrassing remarks in front of everyone else at the office.*

Step 2: Choosing and clarifying a problem to solve—*I'll tackle all three together since they all involve my working relationship with Nick. I need to deal with this because the stress is hurting my family relationships and affecting my mood and health. But I can't believe a guy like Nick is going to be able to hear my complaints objectively and then be willing to change his behavior. What's the use? I'll probably only end up getting a bad performance review if I try to talk to him.*

Step 3: Brainstorming solutions—*(1) Quit immediately. (2) Put up with things as they are. (3) Talk to Nick's supervisor. (4) Have a talk with Nick directly.*

Step 4: Narrowing down the possibilities—*I'm not as powerless as I've been thinking (must be the exhaustion talking): I have total control over my personal life, and I don't have to put up with bullying or oppression at work. It would be tempting to go over Nick's head just to avoid him, but that might just antagonize him further, so I guess I'm going to have to talk to him directly. Bonnie [wife] and Ed [best friend] agree.*

Step 5: Developing and carrying out an action plan—*Here's where my assertive communication skills are going to be central.*

written. When Mike found himself showing more and more of the telltale signs of stress, he decided he needed a Plan B for dealing with Nick's unpleasantness. Given that he'd had little success in changing Nick's behavior once before, what could he do to manage these stressful circumstances?

As Mike's priority list (pages 222–223) showed, his next step was to see if he could reduce his stress by looking at the situation differently. When he examined his thinking

Confront Your Boss or Go Over His Head?

When you're under a lot of stress, bearding the lion in his den doesn't seem very appealing. But consider the pros and cons: While it might initially feel satisfying to go over his head, will you worry later about his finding out? Will the higher-up accurately represent you and your concerns? And how assertive is it to "tattle" on the person who is supervising you directly? In contrast, although there's a small risk he'll resist, confronting your boss about a problem (using nonconfrontational assertive language) is a faster and more up-front route to the results you want. There's no middleman to worry about, you might gain points for having courage, and you'll get practice in communicating effectively.

EYE PENER

Communicating Assertively with Authority Figures

If you have a boss (or, for that matter, a professor if you're in school) who treats you in ways you don't like, you have the right to stand up to this person; just make sure you're respectful of his or her rights as well as your own. In other words, *be assertive*. Here are some things to keep in mind:

1. **Don't rush in.** It's critical that you keep your cool in these situations, and the best way to do that is to let yourself calm down for a little while before marching in. How long? Maybe an hour, maybe a few hours, maybe a day. What's more important is not to complain to friends while you're simmering down—that adds fuel to the fire. Instead, use cognitive therapy techniques to strike your awfulizing and "I can't stand it" thoughts. Remind yourself that you're bigger than this. You can handle it. Tell yourself the anger isn't yours—it's his.

2. **Show respect.** It's okay to disagree with your boss; just make sure it's clear that you respect his position of authority. For example, "I know you're the boss, but I feel I deserve recognition for the ideas that I come up with" or "Nick, I understand that the deadlines are up to you, but I can't be expected to meet them if I don't have any notice that they're being moved up." Putting it this way reduces the intimidation factor and increases the chances of your getting what you want.

3. **Have the evidence.** Write a list of specific examples of what the person did that you didn't like and how it made you feel. Then rehearse and be ready to cite examples on the spot. Maybe she'll become more aware of her behavior and try to control it.

patterns, he recognized a number of common stress-provoking cognitions. Mike listed these in the worksheet on the next page. For practice with changing your own stress-provoking thoughts, use the material in Chapter 8 to identify the type of thinking pattern each of Mike's listed cognitions represents. Then use the cognitive therapy strategies to challenge these cognitions and change them into more helpful, productive, and less stressful ways of thinking. Complete the far right column of the worksheet with new, stress-reducing thinking patterns (the first one is already done as an example).

Changing his thinking patterns helped Mike look at Nick's behavior in a different light. He stopped *demanding* that Nick end his bullying and appreciated that at least he'd been helpful with the workload issues—in other words, *things could be worse*. Mike also realized his own strength in being able to put up with Nick's unpleasant behavior. He even had a hunch that Nick behaved so miserably because he had his own personal problems. While none of this actually changed Nick's behavior, Mike found it a little easier to let it roll off his back. He was even able to view some of it as humorous, something he and his coworkers laughed about and bonded over at happy hour after work. And with his new thinking patterns, Mike was able to keep it together at home too.

HELPING MIKE CHANGE STRESS-PROVOKING THOUGHTS

Stress-*provoking* cognition	Type of thinking pattern	Stress-*reducing* cognition
Nick shouldn't treat me like this. Bosses must treat their workers with respect.	Musturbation (demandingness)	I'd prefer that Nick treat me respectfully, but there's no law that he must; and I can't really control what he does. These are just my preferences.
I can't stand working here if Nick is my boss.		
Nick is ruining my entire life.		
Things will never get better.		
Nick is a terrible person.		

Still, dealing with Nick's aggravating and inconsiderate behavior—even on an occasional basis—was stressful for Mike because of how unpredictable it was. Mike never knew what to expect: Would Nick steal his next great idea? Was he talking about Mike behind his back? Mike found himself becoming more and more suspicious, apprehensive, and even paranoid at work. Since changing cognitions doesn't change the situation (or the *person*) Mike decided he should apply more stress-management techniques. In the worksheet on the facing page, fill in some additional ideas for how he could use the remaining strategies from Part II to manage his stress over Nick's unpredictable behavior.

Find allies at work. Just knowing you've got a coworker who's there to support you, talk about your situation, or help you find humor in it can reduce your stress level.

HOW MIKE COULD MANAGE THE STRESS OF HAVING AN UNPREDICTABLE BOSS

Healthy eating, exercise, and sleep:

Relaxation and meditation:

Time management:

THE RIGHT WORK BUT THE WRONG JOB?

Luis had landed a great job right after graduating with a degree in environmental engineering. The firm he was working for was on the cutting edge of environmentally friendly building design, especially public buildings like schools and libraries. He was making more money than any of his classmates, and if he stuck it out, he'd probably make a name for himself in the field in a few short years. So why was he going home with a massive headache every day? How come he got sleepy at lunchtime and just wanted to go home and nap? Why did he find himself wanting nothing more than to have a drink and be left alone after work?

Luis ended up full of muscle tension before he got into work in the morning because the job seemed great, but it actually wasn't for him. He knew the problem had to be his job, but he kept telling himself that he had no right to complain since a lot of his friends would kill for a job with these perks and this opportunity for advancement. His parents bragged to their friends about their successful son, and his boss often reminded him that he was getting in on the ground floor of something big. How could he stay where he was without losing his mind and his health?

Luis had a strong sense that the statements he was making to himself about what he had to do didn't gibe with his feelings about what he wanted to do, which was quit. So he turned to Chapter 8 to examine his thinking and found he was guilty of an awful lot of *mus*turbation, black-and-white thinking, and jumping to conclusions. Ultimately he realized the environment meant a lot to him, but sitting in front of a computer all day was smothering him. He had always been super-sociable and loved nothing better than a good debate. Luis used problem solving (Chapter 5) and cognitive therapy (Chapter 8) to look at his options. He could have tried to make some changes in his current job, but in the final analysis it became obvious that he wanted to advocate for the environment in a hands-on way, not work as an engineer. With a lot of research, he found a job as an advocate for a nonprofit environmental organization where he could use his engineering knowledge in writing and planning campaigns and his people skills traveling around the country making people aware of the issues at hand. He made less money, but his headaches went away and he felt great about what he was doing.

Tali was a medical student at a very competitive medical school. She'd been working hard, studying nonstop for a couple of years, and knew this was the only way to get ahead. But as she watched her classmates surging ahead of her, getting the best internships, fellowships, and jobs, she had to ask herself why she'd fallen to the back of the pack. She turned to Chapter 1 to take a close look at how the stress was affecting her and realized her physical health was suffering badly, and it showed: she was far too exhausted, she looked pale, she became irritable, she had gained weight from eating whatever she could grab between classes, labs, and studying, and forgoing exercise, and now felt sluggish too. Was medical school worth all this? She had to admit that she could understand why the faculty didn't have much confidence that she'd be able to call up the energy and focus needed to succeed as a doctor. She talked to her supervisor about her problem, and it was instantly clear that she needed to take measures to better manage her time and get control over her health habits—or else the 3 years she'd invested in medical school would be lost. Tali used time management strategies (Chapter 7) to figure out ways to be more efficient and cut down on procrastinating so that she could work more exercise into her life. She signed up at the university fitness center, where she got a trainer to give her some tips on how to exercise. She also started cooking for herself and eating healthier rather than just grabbing fast food or whatever she could find in the library snack machine (Chapter 10). Within a few weeks, Tali was feeling better physically and sleeping better. She was able to spend more time enjoying herself, which made it easier to sit down and study when she needed to. By the end of that semester, the medical school faculty felt so much better about Tali's performance that they'd started referring to her as the "comeback kid."

Max loved his work but just couldn't seem to fit in with his coworkers. He was older than they were, quieter, and in his opinion, a lot more humble. They were, to him, a brash, loud bunch and he couldn't figure out how to talk to them. For their part, his coworkers looked at him as if he were an alien creature and, after lots of failed attempts to start a conversation, they usually kept their distance. What should he do? Try harder to get along with them, get used to being an outsider, or look for a new job? He needed to use the worksheets in Part I of this book to figure out exactly what was bothering him most, how much it bothered him, and what he really wanted. Max eventually figured out that he was quieter than a lot of people and so found a job in a much smaller office where everyone essentially kept their business and personal lives separate. The pressure was relieved at work, and he chose his own social life after he got home.

If you're feeling stressed out at work and yet on the surface it seems as if you have a good job with a fair boss, interesting work, decent income, and reasonable hours, it might take some digging to figure out exactly what the problem is. Don't fall prey to stressful thinking patterns like *shoulds* and *musts* that say you have to stay in a work setting that anyone else would think was a great job. Use the worksheets in Parts I and II of this book to figure out what's really stressing you out, how much, and what would relieve the stress. To help you begin, here's a checklist of signs and symptoms of excessive work (and school) stress. Check the boxes next to any that you're experiencing.

- ❑ Anxiety, irritability, depressed feelings

- ❑ Loss of interest in work (or school)

- ❑ Problems with your sleep

- ❑ Consistently feeling tired in the middle of the day (fatigue)

- ❑ Trouble concentrating

- ❑ Headaches

- ❑ Stomach problems and problems with your appetite

- ❑ Social withdrawal

- ❑ Constantly feeling irritated and then taking it out on important people in your life

- ❑ Reduced sex drive

- ❑ Using alcohol or drugs to cope

Don't ignore these warning signs; they can lead to larger issues as well as physical and emotional health problems. If you can't put your finger on what's causing them, try the exercises in Chapter 5, which teach you how to identify possible problem areas.

PERFORMANCE ANXIETY

Having to perform in front of others, whether it's speaking to a group of people or doing something else while you're being watched, is a significant source of stress for many people in the workforce, especially if you've got what psychologists call *social anxiety disorder*—the extreme fear of embarrassment and tendency to worry about what others think of you. But these kinds of performance situations aren't inherently stressful—it's warped thoughts and beliefs *about* them that cause your anxiety and stress. That's why this is a domain where untwisting a few common mental gremlins is the key to feeling less stressed.

"I'll embarrass myself and it would be *awful!*"

Caryn, who finished her degree and took her first job as an assistant professor in the history department of a university, had social anxiety disorder and found it very stressful to stand up and lecture in front of a large class. What if she posed a question to the class and no one responded? What if they found her class boring? Caryn felt terrified of going to her own classes, losing sleep the night before, and rehearsing exactly what she was going to say. She used the following cognitive therapy strategies: First, she remembered that she'd been embarrassed in the past, but that it wasn't as awful as she'd anticipated. Then she told herself that anything negative that happened in class she could actually use to her *advantage*. For instance, if she asked a question and no one raised their hand to answer, or if students fell asleep in class, she could use it as an amusing story to entertain her family and friends. She also knew that this sort of thing happened to her colleagues, so it wouldn't be personal. Once she realized that nothing permanently catastrophic could happen in class, Caryn was less stressed about teaching. But she still occasionally felt a surge of panic before class at the beginning of a term, when she knew the material would be different and all the students unfamiliar. So she got in the habit of doing progressive relaxation before her classes when she felt panic rise and she had 15 minutes before the class began. If she had only 5 minutes, she used the time to do some diaphragmatic breathing (see Chapter 9). The combination of mental and physical "weapons" really helped, and by

> *A good way to develop trust in your ability to perform in front of others is to practice putting yourself in the spotlight again and again. Start with situations where the stakes are lower (such as having family and friends observe you) and move up to more threatening settings.*

EYE PENER

Shame-Attacking Exercises

Want proof that being embarrassed isn't awful or terrible and that its effects aren't permanent? Follow the advice of the late psychologist Dr. Albert Ellis. He'd have his patients purposely humiliate themselves once a day to learn how not to be ashamed. Ellis's "shame-attacking exercises" included things like purposely spilling food, drink, or a handful of coins in a crowded place, calling out the floors as you ride on a crowded elevator, asking for directions to the place where you're standing, not having enough money to pay for items you bring to the cashier at a store, asking someone for the time when you're clearly wearing a watch, and ordering food that the restaurant obviously doesn't serve (like pizza in an ice-cream parlor). Practicing these therapeutic exercises will teach you that feeling embarrassed doesn't have to be so stressful.

her second year as a teacher she found she was often looking forward not just to reading papers, but to delivering lectures.

"Everyone will notice how anxious and stressed I am."

This cognition makes you feel even *more* anxious and stressed because it provokes the fight-or-flight response and makes you feel as if everyone's paying attention to you. And research shows that people who stress out performing in front of others assume that how they feel inside is exactly how they must look to other people. But it's usually a gross exaggeration. Keep the following in mind: Your heart might be pounding—but no one can see inside your chest. You might have a hot flash, but no one can see this either. And while trembling, sweating, flushing, and a shaky voice might be noticeable, the fact is that people just aren't paying as much attention to these kinds of things as you think. And even if they do notice, remember that no one expects perfection.

"I *must* be perfect."

You don't have to perform *perfectly* to succeed, to get a good performance review, and so on. Everyone makes mistakes, and whoever's watching you perform knows it. Take public speaking, for example. You don't need to be brilliant, relaxed, and witty to be a good public speaker. You can make mistakes, tell bad jokes (or none at all), have a funny-sounding voice, and even get tongue-tied, and still succeed. Most people watching or evaluating you are rooting for you to do a good job; but they don't expect perfection.

TEST ANXIETY

Whether you're being evaluated for a job or promotion, getting certified in a new area, or earning credits for continuing education, test taking is a part of life. And taking tests can be stressful since there's always a possibility of failure. Maybe you'll miss out on a promotion, or miss an opportunity to get certified or licensed; or maybe the consequences are more personal—humiliation when your coworkers find out, or mentally berating yourself for not doing as well as expected. Test anxiety affects people in different ways. Do you lose sleep before a test because you're up catastrophizing about what could happen if you failed? Do you become irritable or difficult to be around? Reducing the stress of test taking is all about preparation . . . and about changing the negative beliefs that plague most people with test anxiety.

Planning and Time Management to Reduce Test Anxiety

Learn about the Test

It seems obvious to say that you should find out as much as you can about the topics that will be covered, the number of questions, the format (such as essay or multiple choice), how much time you'll have to take the test, and how it will be scored, but many people get so nervous about tests that they forget they have the right to ask. Also, if possible, get examples of questions so you have a better idea of what to expect.

Organize Your Studying

Use the time management strategies from Chapter 7 to help you develop a schedule for what you're going to study when. Make sure your schedule is manageable and reasonable so that you feel good about working through it. And test yourself to be sure you're really prepared—it will go a long way toward reducing your anxiety that you might not do well.

Stick to your study schedule. If you find yourself procrastinating, it means that you're being affected by stress-provoking thoughts—a common cause of test anxiety.

Take Care of Your Body

Mental functioning, such as your ability to concentrate while studying and taking tests, is affected by your physical health. So make sure you eat well and exercise (Chapter 10) during test time. And try not to disrupt your daily routine too much as this can throw off your body's internal clock. To optimize your memory and concentration, get plenty of sleep—especially the nights right before the test. Pulling "all-nighters" to study is never a good idea, even if you use caffeine to keep you awake. If you notice yourself experiencing muscle tension and other physical signs of stress, remind yourself that this is normal. Then try relaxation strategies (see Chapter 9) to help you calm down. Taking occasional study breaks will also help you unwind. Whether it's socializing with friends or doing an activity you enjoy, breaks help clear your mind and keep you in the proper frame of mind.

Optimize the Test-Taking Environment

You might not be able to control everything that happens when you take the test, but there are things you can do to minimize distractions. Dress comfortably—perhaps in layers so you're ready if the room is hot or cold. Make sure you're on time, but don't arrive too early—sitting around and waiting can be agonizing and cause negative thoughts to creep into your mind. Arriving late will just give you more to stress about. Choose a seat that's away from doors, aisles, and other high-traffic areas; and sit by yourself if you can. Talking to, or watching, other people who might themselves be nervous can increase your own stress level.

Got a test that you're stressed about? In the worksheet on the facing page, list the steps you can take to prepare. Make a copy and keep it handy as a reminder.

TEST PREPARATION

1. What do I know about the test (length, format, etc.)?

2. When and where will I study (dates, times, place)?

3. What materials do I need to study from?

4. What will I do to make sure I'm in good physical and mental shape for the test (what's my sleep and exercise schedule; what will I eat before the test)?

5. What do I know about the test environment, and what can I do to optimize it (what will I wear to the test, what time will I arrive, and so on)?

Identifying and Changing Stress-Inducing Cognitions

Certain thoughts and beliefs turn test anxiety into a negative vicious cycle that's very hard to stop. Like a self-fulfilling prophecy, cognitions such as "I'm no good at taking tests" make you extremely anxious before and during the test itself. Because you're so stressed about taking the test, you get distracted when you try to study and end up being unprepared. What's more, the anxiety saps your concentration during the test itself, and you end up doing poorly—just as you'd feared. This reinforces your stressful thinking (that you're no good at taking tests) and keeps the cycle going like a runaway train.

So the time to deal with the stressful thinking patterns is *before* you begin preparing for the test. Use Chapter 8 to help you identify, challenge, and change your test-related cognitions and begin thinking in healthier, stress-reducing ways that take some of the pressure off. Look at the worksheet on the facing page, where I've listed stress-provoking cognitions that I often come across

Job-related anxiety is never higher than when you feel the threat of job loss. If you're stressed out by constant worry that you'll lose your job, or you have lost your job, see Chapter 13, where job loss is covered in depth.

in my own work helping students with test anxiety. Use the challenges I've included for each of these mental gremlins to help you come up with more realistic thinking patterns and write these stress-reducing cognitions in the far right column of the table. Do you have other stressful cognitions about tests that aren't listed here? You can use the blank spaces at the bottom of the table to write in and transform them as well.

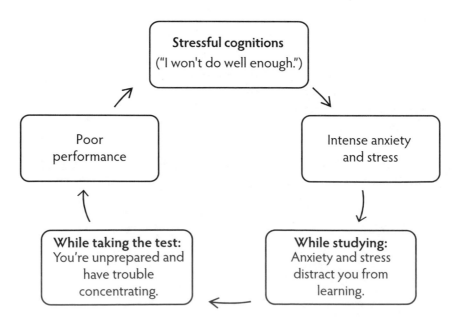

The vicious cycle of test anxiety.

REPLACING STRESS-PROVOKING THOUGHTS
ABOUT TEST TAKING

Stress-*provoking* cognition	Challenges	Stress-*reducing* cognition
I *always* do poorly on tests. I'm just a bad test taker. (extremist thinking and labeling)	Do your past troubles with tests mean this must *always* be a lifelong problem for you? Are you doing *anything* to help yourself (like reading this book!)?	
If I don't pass, I'm a *failure.* (labeling)	Can you *really* sum up who you are with one adjective? Does a single test really determine who you are or what the rest of your life will be like? How will this seem months or years from now?	
I'll *never* learn everything I need to know for the test. (all-or-nothing thinking and jumping to conclusions)	Has your test anxiety hampered your ability to unleash your full studying potential? Do you know for sure that you'll fail? Is it true that you need to know *everything* to pass?	
If I fail this test, my whole life and future will be ruined. (awfulizing)	While failing might be bad, is it truly 101% awful? How will it affect you 5 years from now? What serious injury would you rather have than fail the test?	
I *must* get a good (or *perfect*) grade on every test. (*mast*urbation)	It's *better* to do well, but where is it written that you *must* or *should*? Are you confusing a *desire* with an enforceable decree or law of nature? Are you adding to your stress by putting demands on yourself?	I'd *prefer* to do well on the test, but if I don't . . . (insert other stress-reducing cognitions here)

WORKAHOLISM

☐ Does work seem more exciting than anything else in your life—including your family?

☐ Do you often take work to bed with you?

☐ Do you have trouble staying on time for commitments outside of work because of your work demands?

☐ Has your dedication to work hurt your personal relationships?

☐ Do you think about work while you're talking to others or when on vacation?

If you answer yes to most of these questions, you might be a *workaholic*—the term created to describe someone whose work dominates his or her life to the point that it replaces family, friends, and other outside interests. It's *all* work. Workaholism typically goes with a "Type A" personality, which involves traits such as competitiveness, impatience, and sometimes hostility. Not surprisingly, this personality style is strongly associated with high stress and an increased risk of health problems. The following example of Mia is typical.

> *A hard worker can think about lying on the beach while at work; a workaholic thinks about work while lying on the beach.*

Simply put, Mia worked *too* hard. She was a lawyer—up every morning before dawn and out the door before her husband and children were even awake. She'd come home for dinner on most nights, but usually not until close to the kids' bedtime. Then she'd check in with her husband and get right back to working on the next day's cases. And weekends were often spent holed up in her home office. Mia hadn't attended any parent–teacher conferences, taken any vacations with her family, or spent quality time with her husband in years. And he wasn't pleased with how their marriage was working out. Still, Mia, an excellent lawyer who earned top dollar, was relentless. She took on lots of work at the firm and was very dependable—even if she had to frantically scramble and work to the point of exhaustion to complete projects on time. Mia enjoyed working hard, but also noticed these problems. She was feeling very tired and often felt out of breath. At her last checkup, the doctor even put her on medication for high blood pressure and suggested she stop working so hard, take time to sleep and exercise more, and consider yoga or meditation. The strategies Mia used to combat her workaholism (in addition to changing her sleep and other health habits) can be helpful if you have a similar problem.

Challenging Cognitions in Workaholism

Certain telltale cognitions underlie workaholism and lead to putting work ahead of other important areas of life. It's useful to examine these thoughts and beliefs and modify them into more healthy and realistic (stress-reducing) ways of thinking. The worksheet on the next page lists Mia's stress-inducing cognitions—they're pretty typical. Based on what you learned in Chapter 8, use the challenges to come up with stress-reducing cognitions. Use the blank spaces at the bottom of the worksheet to write in and transform your own stressful cognitions.

Challenging these thinking patterns can help you get a new perspective on your relationship with work—as it did for Mia. And that *might* be enough to help you change your behavior. I'll show you some specific strategies for battling workaholism in just a bit.

Sometimes, however, changing your thinking doesn't lead to changing your behavior. Like many people who work too much, Mia enjoyed working and found it satisfying. In fact, when she was honest with herself, she could admit that throwing herself into her work sometimes seemed more enjoyable than spending time with her family, socializing with friends, relaxing with a good book, taking trips with her husband, and the like. Do you ever feel this way? If so, you might have cognitions such as "I can't stand not working" and "I'm just wasting my time if I'm not getting any work done." These beliefs will compel you to work more and more and make you frustrated when you're not working. And this will disrupt your relationships and keep you from enjoying leisure time—a recipe for long-term stress and related physical problems.

But the truth is that spending time away from work won't kill you. You *can* stand it. And sometimes it's important to make sacrifices—whether for children who look up to you, a spouse or partner who depends on your help and desires your attention, or your own long-term health. If working is very enjoyable for you—maybe even more enjoyable than these other things—that might be difficult to change. But either way, life will be less stressful if you can cut back on working (even a little bit) and diversify your routine, even if you're just going through the motions to please significant others in your life. Here are some strategies for gradually easing up on the amount of time you spend working.

Manage Your Time

If you're a workaholic, chances are managing your time is not your strong suit. Mia used the time management strategies in Chapter 7 to help weaken her addiction to work. In her calendar, she made sure to schedule time for her family every day. Research suggests that you need to spend at least 20 minutes of uninterrupted time with someone on most days to maintain a healthy relationship. She also scheduled at least one half-day activity (such as a hike, trip to the amusement park, or sporting event) with her children per week and one "date night" with her husband every week. No cell phones or PDAs allowed! Mia also enrolled in a cooking

Gradually cut down the number of hours you work each day or week. For example, start with not working on one of the weekend days and take it from there.

CHALLENGING MIA'S WORKAHOLIC THOUGHTS

Stress-*provoking* cognition	Challenges	Stress-*reducing* cognition
I must be perfect. (<u>mus</u>turbation)	Is anyone really perfect? Where is it written that I *must* be? What's a more realistic goal?	
If something isn't flawless, then it isn't worthwhile. (all-or-nothing thinking)	Must my work be *absolutely flawless* to be excellent? What would I say to someone else who told me this?	
I can't be satisfied unless I'm the best—number one. (all-or-nothing thinking)	How do you define the best? The best at what? And what's wrong with being "one of the best"—or "outstanding"? What's really most important here?	
Succeeding at work defines my worth as a person. (labeling)	Is it really that simple? Is work really the only thing that defines me? Work is important, but what about being a parent, a spouse, a friend?	

class—something she'd wanted to take up but never had the time—that met one night each week.

What can you do to manage your time better? Use the strategies in Chapter 7 to develop a plan. Describe your ideas here: _____

_____

_____

_____

Just Say No

It's an essential skill for reducing the time you spend working and getting out from under mounds of requests, assignments, and other work that you don't enjoy (or don't get paid for doing). If you're concerned you'll offend or anger others, review the section on assertiveness in Chapter 6. You can stand up for yourself, your time, and your priorities and still show respect for the person to whom you're saying no. And you don't need to say no to *everything*. In fact, there are probably some requests you're better off saying yes to at work (or school). Here are some practical strategies that Mia used to say no in her work as a lawyer.

Say Yes before You Say No

Think of this as a verbal tennis game. First, say yes to the request. Second, hit the ball back into the other person's court by saying you're overcommitted right now and don't have the time, or by using some other delay tactic. For example, a client asked Mia to read over a contract for one of the client's friends who was renting an apartment. Mia replied, "Sure, but I'm working on preparing for some upcoming cases this month. Can it wait until next month?" When a colleague asked if he could refer a complex legal case to Mia—a case she knew would be exhausting—Mia said, "Thanks for the referral. Would you please set up a meeting with you, me, and the client in a few weeks so we can talk about the details?" These strategies reduced Mia's workload—at least for the time being—without her ever having to use the word "no."

Postpone

With this strategy you don't say yes or no, but instead defer your answer. One of Mia's law partners, for example, asked if Mia would mind editing the firm's training manual for interns. She replied, "My plate is really full right now. Can you ask me again in a few weeks?" Some requesters will make a note to themselves and follow up—but most won't. And if you defer twice in a row, even fewer will ask a third time. If you are asked a third time, however, it's probably a good idea to give a definitive answer (yes or no), rather than keep deferring.

Anticipate

If you feel you're going to be asked to do extra work, make it known that you're very busy before the request is made. For example, at a staff meeting, Mia told her colleagues, "Before we start, I have to let you know that I don't have any room for more clients right now." This served as a warning to the senior partner and ensured that Mia couldn't be blamed if she said no to taking on another case.

Can you think of, or anticipate, requests that you should turn down? Use the space below to write down your strategy. What request will you decline? What will you say?

_____

_____

_____

Increase Your Social Interactions

Mia worked harder to make time to be with friends and to keep her relationships fresh outside her family. She accepted more invitations to "girls' night out" with neighbors and to block parties and used social networking to reconnect with some of her old friends from high school, college, and law school. It made Mia feel good to think back to those times in her life. What are some things you can do to enhance your social life?

_____

_____

_____

Turn Off Your Personal Electronic Devices

Are you so addicted to your cell phone or e-mail that you think you've got to be accessible all the time? Do you obsessively check texts and e-mails and then feel compelled to answer them? Try leaving your electronic devices at home, or just turning them off when you're out of the office, socializing, or on vacation. If you've absolutely got to be reachable, check your phone, texts, or e-mail once an hour (or perhaps less often). You might feel anxious about being out of touch at first, but before too long, you'll see how freeing this can be; and you'll find it's easier to relax than you'd thought.

Be Patient, but Don't Give Up

Mia found that taking the preceding steps wasn't as easy as she'd thought. At times she felt frustrated and anxious—as if going into withdrawal from cutting back on doing so much work. You might also feel guilty, as if you are letting your company or boss down somehow; or depressed, as if you're less useful, important, or worthwhile. If these emotions linger, use the strategies in Chapter 8 to change these faulty thinking patterns. Working toward a healthy work–life balance is just as important as working toward success at your job. You might even find that your work productivity increases as you take more time to relax and connect with the important people in your life.

PREVENTING BURNOUT

❐ Have you lost interest in your job?

❐ Do you feel exhausted just *thinking about* work?

❐ Do daily activities that used to inspire you now seem dull, boring, or mind-numbing?

❐ Have you become more pessimistic and cynical?

❐ At work, does it feel like you're just going through the motions?

If your answer to some of these questions is yes, you might be suffering from burnout or "burnout syndrome"—a state of sheer physical and emotional exhaustion in which you lose interest in your work and career. Daily activities—even those you once found stimulating—start to seem tedious, boring, and overwhelming. Lots of factors may contribute to burnout: working long hours with little down time, a continually stressful work (or school) environment, constant surveillance or inspections by peers or managers, little or no reward or recognition for hard work, unpleasant social circumstances, lack of control over your future, and feeling like nothing you do really makes a difference or is appreciated. And research shows that certain people are particularly at risk: those who feel they must always prove themselves, and those who often neglect their own needs, who tend to deny their own problems, or respond to stress by isolating themselves and using drugs or alcohol. Fortunately, you can use many of the techniques in this workbook to prevent or alleviate burnout. This section describes how.

General Preventive and Treatment Strategies

Keeping a healthy diet, getting frequent exercise, and maintaining good sleep habits are all excellent ways to help prevent burnout. These ensure that you're on top of your game mentally and help you cope with adversity on the whole. Using superior communication skills to help you maintain strong relationships with relatives, friends, and coworkers is also important because it ensures that you have a social support base if needed. Being able to connect with like-minded people makes it easier for you to relax and counter burnout effectively. If conflicts are interfering with some of your important relationships, brush up on your assertiveness and problem-solving skills so you can address these issues productively. Finally, being able to put your body and mind at ease using relaxation and meditation will help you gather your forces and prepare to prevent or take on burnout in the midst of a stressful work or school environment.

EYE OPENER

Recovering from Burnout

What if you're already past the breaking point and it's too late to *prevent* burnout? Trying to fight through the exhaustion and continue as if nothing's wrong will only cause more emotional and physical turmoil. While the strategies for preventing burnout can still be helpful, *recovery* requires these further steps:

- **Burnout recovery strategy #1: Take a time-out.** A full-blown case of burnout is probably not going to be solved by trying to change your thinking, meditating, or exercising more. You need to force yourself to seriously slow down and take a break. In sports, players and coaches use a time-out to strategize about how to beat their opponent. You need to do the same. Cut back on any activities and commitments that you can. Give yourself time and permission to rest, reflect, and regroup.

- **Burnout recovery strategy #2: Stay connected.** When you're burned out, it's natural to want to isolate yourself and cut off ties with family and friends. But you need these people more than ever during difficult times. Don't be afraid to fall back on your loved ones for support. Simply connecting by sharing your thoughts and feelings with someone who cares can help lift some of the load off your shoulders.

- **Burnout recovery strategy #3: Reexamine your goals and priorities.** Burnout is a sure sign that something important in your life isn't working out. So take the opportunity to reflect honestly on your personal desires, dreams, and aspirations. Are you overlooking something that's really important to you? Burnout can be an opportunity to rediscover what makes you happy and to change your life's course accordingly.

Specific Suggestions

Be Assertive at Work

Often some type of organizational change is necessary to prevent or alleviate burnout. For example, if your job has gotten too monotonous, you might need to speak up to a boss or supervisor and assertively ask for different duties. In other instances, you might feel overwhelmed because it's not clear what's expected of you in your job. Here you can use assertiveness skills to meet with a manager and clarify your job description. Having a clear expectation of duties is often of great help in alleviating feelings of burnout. Where do you feel you could be more assertive about making changes to your job?

_____

_____

_____

_____

Keep the Environment Interesting

Try to make being at work more fun or interesting. Could you talk to that new employee you've been meaning to meet? How about playing soft music in the background? Are there tasks you enjoy that you could spend more time with? Try to complete tasks that you don't enjoy right away so that you don't have to spend the whole day dreading having to do them. If there's really nothing at all that you enjoy about your job, your problem might not be burnout, but that you actually need a new job.

Keeping to the same routine day in and day out can quickly lead to boredom. So create job diversity for yourself; for example, ask to change your start time, redecorate or reorganize your workspace, and ask to take on new job tasks. Make sure you're not just taking on more busy work; ask for new assignments you think you'll enjoy. Meanwhile, be creative. Think about how you could modify your current tasks or improve them in a creative way. Take your creative ideas to your supervisor and tell him or her that they may increase productivity or save the company money. Think about ways to combat burnout by making things more interesting at work. Write your ideas here:

_____

_____

_____

TAKING STOCK: YOUR "INTERNAL AUDIT"

As most vocational counselors would recommend, it's a good idea to occasionally take stock (once or twice a year) of your job or career—even when things seem to be going well—just to see if there's any stress building up in the background, or minor problems you could address to prevent your stress from increasing. This "internal audit" might be as simple as asking yourself what, if anything, you might change about the work you're doing, the working environment, and so on. You might assess how much time you're devoting to work versus leisure, family, and other non-work-related activities to make sure you've got a work–life balance that's working for you. Finally, take the time to examine your sleeping habits, eating, and exercise patterns. Do you notice any of the physical problems associated with stress? If things seem to be going well, then you're probably managing the normal work stressors well. But better to know this, or to identify any possible signs of too much stress, than be caught off guard.

12

Managing Relationship and Family Stress

Laurie gets home from work hoping to relax, unwind, and just spend some quiet time with her family. Yet the house is anything but quiet and relaxing. The kids need help with homework, there are bills to pay, and decisions to discuss with her husband, Dean, who never seems to be in the mood to talk. This isn't how Laurie envisioned family life. In fact, sometimes it seems like going to work is less stressful then being at home, which is why Laurie has started staying at work later and later each evening. When she is at home, she's tense, irritable, and has heart palpitations. She has a short fuse with her kids and with Dean. Laurie's sleep has suffered too.

Every year, Marty, his wife, Ellen, and their three kids travel across the country to be with Ellen's family for the holidays. But every year it's the same story. Ellen's mother critiques Marty's professional and financial decisions and even how they're raising their kids. To make matters worse, Marty's father-in-law and brother-in-law bait him into the same heated political discussion that turns into personal attacks on Marty because of his different stance on social issues. Before long, Marty's wondering why he even goes to the trouble to travel so far to visit his in-laws when all they do is put him down.

Let's face it: as Laurie's and Marty's stories illustrate, no one can quite get under your skin like the members of your own family. And if you feel like some of your most stressful times are those you spend with your loved ones, you're not alone. It's entirely normal. But there's a good explanation: You expect a lot from your family members—and they expect a lot from you. And neither you nor they can fulfill these expectations all the time. Understanding this is the first step toward better managing relationship and family stressors.

YOUR RELATIONSHIP AND FAMILY STRESSORS

What (or *who*) are the sources of relationship or family stress in your life? Some of them might be obvious to you: Do you and your spouse argue a lot? Are you going through a separation or divorce? Is there a relative you can't stand to be around? Maybe you get stressed out by the holidays. Perhaps your evolving views on politics, religion, or child rearing have led to a falling-out in your family. Perhaps you've got a child who's having real problems in school.

But there could also be more subtle stressors. Do you still feel that you must always please your parents or gain their approval even though you're an adult? Maybe it seems like you're in competition with a sibling for your mom or dad's favor. Maybe you feel like you have to be the ideal friend or the perfect neighbor. Or you spend hours planning or getting ready for every date and then have no fun at all because you're busy trying to figure out whether this new candidate will turn out to be your soul mate. Your personal beliefs and expectations can play a huge role in family and relationship stress. Many of us demand more of ourselves than we'd dream of asking of anyone else. Or we hold both ourselves and those who have an important place in our lives to extremely high standards. Do you *expect* your spouse or partner to be totally devoted and approve of everything you say and do? Do you *insist* that your kids be straight-A students? Do you *demand* that your home be immaculate all the time every day? Do you *count on* your relatives to always be considerate, keep their promises, help you in a pinch, and behave themselves at family gatherings? Chances are you wouldn't use such rigid terms in verbalizing your relationship expectations. But when it comes to negotiating life with valued others, we often lean a little farther toward absolutes and zero tolerance than we realize. Maybe we want to be perfect in the eyes of those we care about so they'll keep us around. And maybe we strike a silent bargain that they, in turn, will fulfill all our expectations. These, after all, are the people we care about most. These are the people who are supposed to have our back. Whatever the case may be, the first step in reducing the stress of relationships is often to recognize these thoughts and feelings. Doing so can help you turn aside potential problems before the stress they cause gets out of hand.

Imperfection is a fact of life, and trying to perfect other human beings and your relationships can become a huge source of stress. If, instead of agonizing over how you can get someone to change a behavior or characteristic you find difficult to take, you told yourself just to accept it as part of this person, how would you feel, think, and/or act differently? What might happen to your stress over this issue?

So, think about what's got you stressed about your relationships, and in the blanks at the top of the next page, list your most stressful events, situations, feelings, and thoughts. If you're having a hard time identifying these, use the My Problem Cues worksheet from Chapter 5 (page 86) to help you identify problem stressors.

Let go of the belief that your home should be a place of rest and tranquility. And give up the idea that family gatherings should be completely free from stress. Though you love your

---

MY SOURCES OF RELATIONSHIP AND FAMILY STRESS

1. _____

2. _____

3. _____

4. _____

5. _____

6. _____

7. _____

---

family and want to enjoy spending time with them, your relatives can be a significant source of stress. Here are some of the most common sources of family and relationship stress:

1. Divorce/stepparent situations

2. Insufficient income

3. Uncooperative children

4. A child with medical or psychological problems

5. A child with poor grades

6. Lack of communication among family members

7. Inflexibility of a spouse or partner

8. Sexual problems between partners

9. Excessive spending by a partner

10. Disagreements with parents, siblings, or other relatives over important family matters (for example, how to handle arrangements after a death in the family)

Luckily, you can take steps to quell your stress over family and relationship matters. In this chapter you'll learn how to apply strategies from Part II of this workbook to address a number of relationship and family stressors.

RELATIONSHIP PROBLEMS AND BREAKUPS

Stress comes with the territory when you're in a close relationship—no matter how sweet your marriage or partnership might be. In fact, half of adults who suffer from severe stress blame at least some of it on their spouse or partner: "He has no time for me now that we're together." "She doesn't understand me." "All he does is work and watch sports on television." "She spends too much money." But the truth is that everyone has a good side and a bad side—there are things we love about our partner and things we dislike. In this section, you'll learn how to apply stress management techniques to help you cope with three aspects of relationships: your partner's annoying behavior, full-blown disagreements or conflicts, and breakups.

Annoyances

Like everyone else, you have ideas or "rules" about how people should behave. And when your partner or spouse violates these rules, it can seem anywhere from annoying to downright maddening. Your muscles become tense, your heart races, maybe you seethe with anger and tell yourself "He's doing this just to make me mad!" or "She knows I don't like it when she _____!"). In the following spaces, list your spouse or partner's top five annoying behaviors. What does your partner do that really gets under your skin?

Top Five Annoying Behaviors

1. _____

2. _____

3. _____

4. _____

5. _____

Laurie got stressed and irritable when Dean broke some of her rules. For example, on the kitchen counter Laurie kept a grocery list that she would use for the family food shopping each week. She'd probably reminded Dean more than 100 times in their 15 years of marriage to write on the list anything they ran out of so she'd know to buy more the next time she went shopping. Laurie's rule was this: *if it's not on the grocery list, it won't be bought*. What really got under Laurie's skin was when Dean would say (as he helped her unpack the groceries), "Where's the coffee? We're out of coffee, you know." "No," she would say, seething. "How would I know? *You* make the coffee in the morning, and *you* didn't add coffee to the list."

Can you put yourself in Laurie's place? Better yet, think of your own reaction when your loved one does something on your list from page 246. What would make Laurie (and you) less stressed? Exploding in anger to get your point across better? Ignoring the behavior, hoping it goes away? Maybe it would help to calmly explain how angry you feel. Perhaps analyzing and changing the way you think about these behaviors would reduce your stress as well?

Here's a list of the stress management techniques you learned about in Part II. Which of these do you think are best suited for managing stress over a loved one's annoying behavior? Rank them in order by inserting a number in the blank to the left of those you favor (1 for first choice, 2 for second, and so on). For those strategies you feel might help, briefly describe in the blank to the right how you'd implement them.

_____ Problem solving: _____

_____ Communication/assertiveness: _____

_____ Time management: _____

_____ Cognitive therapy: _____

_____ Muscle relaxation: _____

_____ Meditation: _____

_____ Healthy lifestyle: _____

Laurie decided to use assertiveness and cognitive therapy. She held out some hope of changing Dean's behavior (through assertiveness), but also realized that changing her thinking (cognitive therapy) would make her own stress levels less dependent on Dean's behaving according to her rules. The following section describes what Laurie did.

Assertiveness

Laurie didn't like putting up with Dean's annoying behavior and felt she could be more assertive with him. So, working through Chapter 6, she came up with the following assertive statement, which she said calmly yet firmly when Dean asked her why she hadn't thought to buy something that he didn't put on the grocery list: "Dean, I've reminded you over and over that if you want me to buy something, you have to write it on the grocery list. Thank you for listening." And instead of stomping out the door in anger to return to the store, when her husband asked where the coffee or other item was, she'd calmly explain, "I'm sorry, Dean, but you didn't write it down on the grocery list, so I didn't buy it. If you want the coffee, you'll have to go to the store yourself. I have other things to do and don't have time to make a second trip." Sometimes Dean opted to go without coffee for a day, but when he realized that meant Laurie had to start her day without it too, he resolved to add coffee to the list, which he did most of the time. No one's perfect. And when he forgot, he made the extra trip to the store.

Use the strategies you've chosen to manage stress in your intimate relationships, but also when you're feeling aggravated with other family members—such as a brother, sister, aunt, or uncle—and close friends. Here are some examples. What strategies would you use with . . .

- Your brother, who promises to help plan your parents' birthday celebration and chip in for a present—and never does?

  _____

  _____

- Your aunt, who still calls you "Pudge" and passes around pictures of you as a chubby child at every holiday?

  _____

  _____

- Your mother-in-law, who tsk-tsks about your kids' low grades, poor manners, or bad habits within earshot of them every time she comes over?

  _____

  _____

- Your best friend, who reveals your secrets and then acts like you're overreacting when you protest?

  _____

  _____

Of course, with assertiveness, there's no guarantee anything you do is going to change the other person's behavior, even if you stick to your guns like Laurie did. But changing the person's behavior doesn't need to be the goal in cases like these. Instead, just aim not to let the other person's behavior add to your stress level. That's what Laurie did when she refused to go back to the store

Cognitive Therapy

Laurie knew she'd better have a back-up plan for managing stress if and when assertiveness didn't work. That's why she also turned to cognitive therapy. Using what she learned in Chapter 8, Laurie discovered that she had the following cognitions about Dean and the grocery list:

> *Your spouse or partner is more likely to change annoying behavior when you refuse to make it your problem and instead make it his or her problem.*

- My grocery list is the only way I can keep track of what we need; therefore Dean should use it.

- Dean should take my advice for being more efficient.

- Dean is being disrespectful to me if he doesn't use the grocery list.

- Dean's forgetfulness is going to get our family in trouble with much more serious matters than groceries. So he just has to get his act together.

Laurie's expectations of Dean—that he *must* follow her rules and advice for being efficient, otherwise he was disrespectful and would lead the family into ruin—seem pretty exaggerated when they're written down. You can probably see how these beliefs led Laurie to become angry and take it personally when Dean didn't use the grocery list even though it seems like a pretty minor matter.

When Laurie analyzed her thinking, she recognized that although the grocery list was efficient, she couldn't control whether Dean actually complied with it—and *expecting* or *demanding* that he *always* take her advice would only lead to becoming angry if and when he didn't. Laurie also realized that, even though she thought Dean was deliberately being disrespectful in not complying with her wishes, she was engaging in *mind reading* since she couldn't be certain about Dean's intent. In fact, there were many times when he *did* use the grocery list. And Laurie also realized that labeling Dean as dangerously forgetful was probably an exaggeration (awfulizing). The fact that he sometimes forgot to add items to the grocery list didn't mean he was going to forget to mail their income tax return or refill their son's asthma medication.

Thinking this through helped Laurie take a new perspective when Dean didn't use the grocery list (or follow some of her other "rules" around the house): "Although I really wish Dean would take my advice when it comes to being more efficient, I can't control his every behavior. Everyone forgets things sometimes, makes mistakes, or acts against their best interest. Dean is usually responsible when it comes to the important things in our lives. He doesn't mean any disrespect." At first it seemed foreign to Laurie to try to think like this. Was she simply letting Dean off the hook? But soon she realized that although these new cognitions didn't solve all of her problems, they were more reasonable than her expectations that Dean do exactly as she wanted when she wanted. Laurie kept an index card in her pocket that read, "It's just Dean being Dean," which she pulled out and read whenever she felt herself becoming aggravated by something her husband did. In addition to being assertive, reading this little reminder reduced Laurie's frustration (and sometimes even made her chuckle), and before long she noticed herself getting worked up less often and feeling a little more relaxed and in control at home as a result.

Handling Your Own Stressors

Laurie's complaint may seem all too familiar to you. Or you might be wondering why I spent so much time on showing how she could work through what seems like a relatively trivial problem. The fact is that it's these little annoyances that can add up to entrenched resentment and major stress. In fact, research consistently shows that along with financial problems, trouble communicating about everyday "minor" complaints is one of the *major* stressors for many couples.

Now that you've seen how Laurie used assertiveness and cognitive therapy to manage her stress level in response to Dean's annoying behavior, try putting these techniques to work for the annoying behaviors you listed on page 247. Write down your new assertive responses and stress-reducing cognitions in the worksheet below. Laurie's example is there to help guide you. Remember, you can assertively ask for changes, but it's important to accept that your loved one isn't perfect and that you can't expect to be able to control him or her. Sometimes it will be up to you to think differently to help reduce your stress response.

Disagreements and Conflicts

Disagreements and conflicts occur in every relationship—whether it's over big-ticket items like finances (how much money to spend and what to spend it on), children (where to send them to school), and other family issues (whose side of the family to spend the holidays with) or less important issues such as what movie to see tonight or who should do the food shopping this week. But when they happen, they're unsettling. You feel

MANAGING ANNOYANCES

Brief description of the annoyance	Assertive responses (new *thinking* patterns)	Stress-reducing cognitions (new things to *say* and *do*)
Dean asks me why I haven't bought something when he hasn't written it down on the grocery list.	<u>Say</u>: "I've reminded you over and over that if you want me to buy something, you have to write it on the grocery list. Thank you for listening." <u>Do</u>: stop going to the store again.	I wish Dean would use the grocery list, but he doesn't <u>have</u> to. He means no disrespect, but he'll have to learn the hard way. I'm not giving in anymore.

frustration and mental anguish, along with tension and irritability. At some point almost everyone has lost sleep over disagreements with a partner or spouse, a child, or another relative.

Often, your first inclination is to try to prove your point, change your partner's mind, set him or her straight, and get them to see things your way. Take Laurie and Dean's ongoing disagreement over child care duties. Laurie feels Dean should help out more with the kids, but Dean feels that no matter what he does, Laurie will still complain that it's not enough. Both partners walk on eggshells around the topic, avoiding the discussions they need to have to resolve the problem.

What are the areas of disagreement in your relationship? Write them down in the spaces below, and as you read about Laurie and Dean, consider how you'd use the strategies in Part II to help you manage stress over your own disagreements.

_____

_____

_____

_____

Laurie finds Dean watching the ballgame on TV instead of supervising the kids as they get ready for bed. Her blood boils as she thinks, "Not again! Hasn't he learned!?" And she erupts, yelling "What's the matter with you!? You *never* help with the children! You think I should supervise the kids while you just sit around!" Of course, Dean feels defensive; and instead of really listening to Laurie, he's only thinking of how to strike back, such as saying "The kids can get ready for bed by themselves. They don't need me watching everything they do. You're just like my mother. No matter what I do, you're *never* happy!" The argument that ensues only provokes more stress in the couple's relationship.

Flip back to the list of stress management techniques on page 246. What strategies would you suggest Laurie use to reduce her stress when she and Dean disagree over child care? Maybe you've recognized that this requires a two-pronged approach, including (1) effective communication and (2) problem solving. Laurie reviewed the techniques in Chapter 6 and came up with ways to discuss this difficult subject with Dean without being threatening or confrontational. For example, "Dean, I'm upset with you right now. It really hurts my feelings when you're sitting there watching the ballgame and relaxing while I'm cleaning up from dinner, especially after you told me you'd keep an eye on the kids."

Psychologist and relationship expert Donald Baucom recommends using the tips in the box on page 254 when discussing concerns with your spouse or partner (or other close family member). Set ground rules so that both of you use these guidelines to ensure a productive, stress-reducing conversation in which you're taking turns getting your feelings out in the open (review the tips or ground rules in the box together with the

EYE 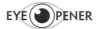 PENER

Discussing Disagreements with Your Spouse or Partner—*Dos* and *Don'ts*

- **Don't say hurtful things.** Saying words you know will hurt your partner's feelings only harms your relationship. Later on, you'll end up regretting and stressing out over what you said. Instead, if you feel the urge to say something hurtful or insulting, say something like "I'm feeling very angry right now. Before I say anything I don't want to, let me cool off." Then take a time-out and use meditation or relaxation techniques from Chapter 10 to help you calm down and collect your thoughts. You can then use the communication skills from Chapter 6 to help you come up with a productive way to continue the conversation.

- **Avoid "kitchen sinking."** This is when you dredge up disagreements and other concerns that happened in the past—perhaps even years ago. It's usually meant to be hurtful and certainly doesn't address the issues right in front of you. Keep the discussion fruitful and civilized by sticking to the matter at hand.

- **Accept some blame.** When you act like you're always right, your partner is less likely to open up to you about what's bothering him or her. Your partner will feel like it doesn't do any good since you think you're always right. So, try to find something specific that you can take blame for. And though it might be hard, say you're sorry *first*—and really mean it. When you admit you're wrong, and then show it with your actions, you demonstrate respect for your partner and he or she will be more willing to forgive and forget.

other person). The purpose of these conversations is twofold: first, to make sure you and your partner understand each other's perspective on the situation; and second, to let each other know you're listening.

You'll be surprised—sometimes, just discussing each others' thoughts and feelings alleviates stress and smooths over disagreements. But if not, the next step is to problem-solve and make decisions about what (if any) changes are needed to resolve the issue. Chapter 5 provides a framework for solving problems and making decisions when disagreements arise, such as over who will handle which household chores, if your family should relocate so your spouse can take a new job, or whether to send your child to public or private school. Laurie and Dean used problem solving to arrive at a solution to their ongoing child care disagreements, which was to plan in advance who would be in charge of the kids at various points through the day. They also agreed that while the kids didn't need to be constantly watched closely (after all, they were 10 and 7 years old), being "on duty" meant being within earshot so that if any problems arose they could be dealt with easily.

Solving problems in a relationship is a little different from solving them on your own since you both need to have input. On the next page are some tips for adapting the problem-solving steps taught in Chapter 5 for when you and your spouse or partner need to solve problems together:

Sharing Thoughts and Feelings to Reduce Stress

Tips for the Speaker

- Emphasize your emotions (how you feel about your partner's actions).

- Give your thoughts and feelings as your own, not as absolute truths.

- Try to include something positive along with your concerns and negative feelings.

- Be as specific as possible.

- Take turns and speak in short paragraphs so that your partner has a chance to respond to one main idea at a time.

- Be tactful so your partner can listen to what you are saying without becoming defensive.

Tips for the Listener

- You don't have to agree with everything your partner is saying, but when he or she is speaking, show that you understand what's being said.

- Put yourself in your partner's shoes and think about the disagreement from his or her angle to help you understand how he or she thinks and feels about the issue.

- When your partner is done speaking, try to summarize his or her most important thoughts and feelings. This shows you've been listening.

- **Don't** ask questions, except for clarification.

- **Don't** interrupt with your own viewpoint or opinion.

- **Don't** change the meaning of your partner's statements.

- **Don't** try to solve the problem.

- **Don't** judge what your partner is saying.

Adapted with permission from Snyder, D. K., Baucom, D. H., and Gordon, K. C. (2007). *Getting Past the Affair.* Copyright 2007 by The Guilford Press.

- **Step 1: Recognizing problems.** Make sure you both agree on the specifics of the problem and that you're both ready to discuss it. State the disagreement in terms of behaviors (for example, "Clark wants Erica to initiate sex more often, but Erica feels this should be her husband's role"), not opinions or labels (for example, "Erica's such a prude").

- **Step 2: Choosing and clarifying a problem to solve.** Explain to your partner what you'd like taken into account when you make a decision—for example, that Clark feels like he has to beg for sex, plus it's a turn-on for him when Erica does make the first move.

- **Step 3: Brainstorming solutions.** Do this together as a team.

- **Step 4: Narrowing down the possibilities.** Go through the possible solutions and choose one that both of you can live with. There might not be a perfect solution, which means both of you should be prepared to compromise. Just make sure both of you feel that the solution you choose is something you'll both actually do without feeling angry or resentful.

- **Step 5: Developing and carrying out an action plan.** Work this out together, too. If applicable, decide on a trial period to evaluate how the solution or decision is working. Don't worry if you have to try out your solution several times before it

---

Resolving Conflicts between Family Members

What about when two (or more) members of your family have disagreements with each other—such as your spouse and one of your children? Arguments among family members can be very stressful for everyone—not just the people involved. And they occur in most families at some point. How you deal with them is often more important than the dispute itself. You can use some of the strategies in Chapter 5 to help you resolve family disputes quickly and fairly. The key is to make sure all involved feel that they're being taken seriously. Here are some tips:

- **Clarify.** First, try to understand the problem or disagreement by having both people involved explain how they feel. This will help you clarify the true source of the argument. For example, Tommy (a seventh grader) wants to enjoy the winter vacation and feels he shouldn't have to do any schoolwork; but Mom feels it's important for Tommy to spend at least an hour every day—even over the holidays—practicing from an algebra workbook she bought for him.

- **Treat others with respect.** As the moderator, make sure you keep this process orderly; otherwise, a good solution will be very hard to find. For example, insist that when one person is talking, the other listens—even if they disagree. Encourage others to understand where each person is coming from. Don't tolerate rudeness or raising voices. For example, Mom should at least listen to Tommy explain how he'd like a break from school for the 2 weeks he has off. Tommy, on the other hand, needs to hear Mom out and understand that she's concerned about Tommy's algebra grade.

- **Brainstorm solutions.** Have everyone involved brainstorm possible solutions together. Make sure each person feels that his or her input is well received. Then review each solution and decide as a group which one to use. Later, get feedback from each person on how the solution is working and how he or she feels about it. In the end, Tommy and his mom came to an agreement that Tommy would use the workbook every other day over the holiday vacation.

feels right. Clark and Erica decided to try scheduling times for sexual rendezvous, including having sex in places other than the bed, and at different times of day, such as while the kids were at school. Both of them found these trysts exciting and satisfying.

Breakups

Whatever the reason, the breakup of a marriage or other long-term, committed relationship is a significant stressor. After all, it represents the loss of companionship, shared dreams, commitments, and intimacy—the failure of a personal connection. Breakups can turn your whole world upside down. Your routine and responsibilities, your home, your relationships with family and friends—all can become disrupted. You might lose your appetite, have trouble sleeping, and even lose the motivation to do things you typically enjoy—hobbies, socializing, work, and so on. And breakups can trigger all sorts of painful and unsettling thoughts and feelings from extreme disappointment to grief to uncertainty and anxiety, anger, and depression. What will it be like without your partner? Will you find someone else? Will you end up alone?

Stress and emotional pain are inevitable in the wake of a breakup. If you've gone through one, your grief, anger, and fear are real. But these emotions become even more intense if you fall into the stressful thinking patterns you learned about in Chapter 8. Labeling and blaming your ex-partner for all the hurtful things he or she did or said to you, for example, intensifies your anger until you're seething. Awfulizing, predicting worst-case scenarios about financial ruin or your children being emotionally scarred for life, makes you more anxious than you need to be. Jumping to conclusions and mind reading, being overly self-critical, and imagining that family and friends will be critical of you and see you as a loser, increases feelings of depression and self-blame.

By now, you've probably guessed that using cognitive therapy to change stress-inducing thoughts and cognitions is one of the best strategies for minimizing the stress of a breakup. For example, when you catch yourself thinking, "I can't stand being alone," replace this with more realistic thinking, such as "I'm surviving, and I can adjust to this new life if I give myself some time and try some new things." Using what you learned in Chapter 8 every day for a little while to help you change these thinking patterns can help you control your stress, let go of the old relationship, and move on. In the worksheet on the facing page you'll find some of the more common breakup-related stress-provoking cognitions along with ways of challenging these mental gremlins. Use these challenges to come up with more realistic thinking patterns that reduce stress and write them in the last column. There's also space for you to write in and work through some of your own stressful cognitions that might be different from those I've already included.

In the aftermath of a difficult breakup it's easy to fall into unhealthy behavior patterns that have a way of developing into a vicious cycle. For example, if you tend to eat in response to stress, your emotional exhaustion and fear of disapproval may lead you to develop unhealthy eating patterns, which can lead to gaining weight and feeling more stressed. Feelings of depression can cause you to withdraw from your social network.

CHALLENGING STRESS-PROVOKING THOUGHTS ABOUT A BREAKUP

Stress-*provoking* cognition	Challenges	Stress-*reducing* cognition
I'm unlovable. (depression)	Is it really true that <u>no one</u> has or will ever love you? Just because <u>your ex</u> doesn't love you anymore, does it really mean that you can't be loved?	
It's my fault. I should have been a better spouse/partner. (depression)	Is it <u>entirely</u> my fault? Doesn't everyone have strengths and limitations? What good does blaming myself do? Did I make mistakes I can learn from?	
I'll never find anyone else <u>or</u> he/she is the only one for me. (anxiety)	Where's the evidence? Am I jumping to conclusions? How do I know what will or won't happen in the future—especially if I get out and meet people?	
People will think I'm a loser. (anxiety)	Am I mind reading? Can I really expect everyone to approve of me all the time? Might some people understand my situation and sympathize with me?	
He/she is a rotten @#%! (anger)	Was my ex 100% rotten? Was there anything I liked about him/her? Were there things I could have done differently?	

EYE 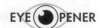 PENER

Being Independent after a Breakup

When a significant relationship ends, feeling good about your identity as an individual can help reduce your stress. Start by taking stock of your strong points, interests, and values. What makes you feel good about being you? Also, try to reclaim that part of yourself that you might have let go during the relationship. For instance, if you quit your band because your partner hated you leaving a couple evenings a week for rehearsals, find a new band to join—or form your own. It can help to share your feelings with someone you trust—but don't become overly dependent on family, friends, or (worse) your ex. Doing so could keep you from getting on with your life and establishing new relationships. Instead, keep yourself busy. Take up a new hobby, redecorate your home, find a new hangout, and so on. And to help you more fully accept your new identity, try mindfulness meditation. Facing the reality that things are different—you're independent—and challenging yourself to explore new interests, activities, and new people will reduce your stress in the present and give you hope for the future.

But if you avoid calling friends and turn down invitations, you'll become isolated and even more stressed. Have you developed any unhealthy or counterproductive behavioral patterns after breaking up? List them below. Use the material in Chapter 10 to help you get back on track with a healthy lifestyle. The Eye Opener above might also be helpful if you're having trouble socializing. Last but not least, many people turn to meditation to help them get back their personal focus.

Behaviors I'd Like to Change Following My Breakup

_____

_____

_____

PARENTING

If you're a parent, then you know that stress is part of your job description. From the time you get up in the morning until the time you collapse into bed at night, you're surrounded by physical and emotional demands. Getting your children up, fed, and off to school on time, then handling homework and after-school activities and dinner, and preparing for bed are physically and mentally draining. Do the daily hassles of this routine—the arguments, squabbling, and dawdling—get to you? Does the pressure build over time? Do you feel your muscles tense with frustration and your fuse become shorter? In the worksheet on the facing page, write down the five most stressful aspects of child care for you. Then think about which of the stress management techniques would be helpful for addressing each area. Refer to the list of techniques on page 248.

Danny and his wife, Sandy, had a second grader, Matt, who was having problems in school learning how to read. He'd fallen far behind the rest of the class and was feeling self-conscious and upset over being "different" from the other students, who it seemed could all read independently. Danny and Sandy felt overwhelmed by Matt's difficulties. They lost lots of sleep worrying about what would become of Matt and what they could do about his learning problems. Would he *ever* learn to read? Would he have to repeat the second grade? Would he need to have a tutor or go to summer school? They worried about how all of this would affect Matt's self-esteem and his future. How would he function in high school? Would he get into a good college? Danny and Sandy found themselves more and more irritable, often snapping at each other, and at Matt, in frustration. On one hand, they wanted to ignore the problem—hopefully Matt would just grow out of it. But every day homework time was a stark reminder that Matt's problem—and their stress—couldn't be left alone any longer.

That's when Danny and Sandy turned to the problem-solving strategies from Chapter 5. Together they came up with a plan that started with scheduling a conference with Matt's teacher. From there, Matt was tested for a learning disability, which led to further recommendations. Danny and Sandy learned that Matt wasn't alone in his struggles with reading (which helped reduce a good deal of their stress) and that there was plenty of help available for him through the school system. It would, however, require lots of time and effort, which is why Sandy turned to the time management techniques in Chapter 7 to help her prioritize and free up more of her schedule to help Matt. Danny did some reading about learning disabilities and applied cognitive therapy techniques (Chapter 8) to help him change his stress-provoking awfulizing cognitions into more realistic

TOP SOURCES OF PARENTING STRESS

Child-related stressors	Stress management techniques
1.	
2.	
3.	
4.	
5.	

EYE 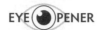 PENER

Make Time for Yourself

To ease the stress of parenting, carve out free-time slots that are not combined with other activities or responsibilities. In other words, make time for yourself that doesn't include the kids. It doesn't make you a bad parent. And it doesn't mean you don't enjoy spending time with your kids. Everyone needs a break once in a while, and spending free time with friends, your spouse, or even alone can help you enrich these relationships and make you appreciate more the time you spend with your children. In the space below, list some activities you can do without your children.

_____

_____

_____

and less stressful ones (such as "Most people with learning disabilities do just fine with accommodations. School might be a struggle, but with the right help, Matt can do just as well as anyone else"). The couple also joined a health club and took up exercising together three times a week to help reduce the physical tension they'd both been feeling. With these changes, Danny and Sandy were able to manage their stress more successfully. What's more, they worked as a team to help Matt as much as they could. Feeling that they were on the right track, they began to sleep better, even after struggling with Matt through long and arduous homework sessions.

Jennifer had it all—a great husband, a high-paying job, a stunning home, and three beautiful and successful children: Taylor (age 18) was an expert skier who had almost made the Olympic team. Cole (age 16) was a near-straight-A student and class president who was destined for Harvard or Yale. And Katie (age 14) was a prima ballerina who got just about every part she auditioned for. So with everything going so well, why was Jennifer's stomach always in knots? Why was she losing sleep at night? Why was she short-tempered all the time? And why did she seem to have headaches every day?

Jennifer was a ball of stress and tension because although things seemed great, they were never great *enough*. Sure, she realized her kids were very successful—she bragged about them to everyone she knew. But her problem was that she could never appreciate her kids' accomplishments because she kept demanding more and more. "I want to be able to tell everyone that you're in the Olympics," she told Taylor. "Your grandparents will be so proud of you when you get into Yale," she'd say to Cole. And "Every girl at school will wish she was you when you get the part of Clara in *The Nutcracker*," she said to Katie. Jennifer's expectations had gone through the roof. And all the pressure she put on her kids was making them very competitive and stressed out as well. They resented their mother's demands. The result was that Jennifer's relationship with her children was suffering—she couldn't enjoy her family—which only added to her stress.

If Jennifer didn't see it, her husband did. And after a lot of coaxing, he finally convinced Jennifer that stress was affecting her and that she needed to take action. Working through Chapter 8 (cognitive therapy) helped Jennifer realize how large a role her thinking was playing in her stress. Stress-inducing beliefs like "People won't think I'm a good parent unless my kids are perfect" and "I've got to have everyone's approval" were two of the main culprits. It wasn't easy (she'd been thinking this way for many years), but Jennifer challenged herself to see the problems with these cognitions and try out more useful, stress-reducing ones, such as "No one is perfect, and people don't expect my kids to be perfect" and "It's just not possible to have everyone's approval all the time." Doing cognitive therapy helped relieve some of the pressure, yet Jennifer still felt strongly that it was important for her kids to be number one—maybe it was her own strict upbringing. But at the same time, she remembered how she wished her own mother hadn't put so much pressure on

> *There are no perfect children—nor perfect parents. Wanting the perfect family can get in the way of enjoying the family you have.*

EYE PENER

Spending Quality Time as a Family

You certainly don't have to do *everything* as a family, but the quality time you *do* spend together helps build family ties to weather all kinds of disputes and stressors. Here are some ways to increase family quality time.

Family projects. Getting the whole family involved in projects and chores in and out of the house increases communication, lightens the workload for each person, and gives everyone a sense of accomplishment and togetherness. It's teamwork that's the essential ingredient here. I'm talking about routine chores, such as doing the dishes together, washing the car, and cleaning the house, and larger projects like spring cleaning and holding a garage sale. Your family could also volunteer together at the local soup kitchen or retirement home.

Eat together. Meals are an ideal time to connect with family members, check in, catch up on everyone's activities, and plan family events. Try to have at least one family meal per day (or *almost* every day). If dinnertime is too hectic at your place, have family breakfasts.

Family events. Special family events can be as easy as a family movie night or outing to the mall, or as elaborate as a family vacation. Whatever the event, find a way to plan it together and give each family member a task that contributes to making it successful and enjoyable. For example, how about a family movie night? Make a list of movies that you all want to see. Then choose one for a specific night. That night, Mom washes the dishes, Emily dries them, Miriam pops the popcorn, and Dad sets up the home theater.

her. So she began easing off on the demands and turned to meditation and exercise to relieve even more of her stress.

FINANCIAL STRESSORS

Finances can be one of the biggest sources of stress in a couple or family's relationship. And these days, as you try to navigate through the struggling economy, financial stress in relationships is at an all-time high. Learning how to put stress management skills to work in this area can mean the difference between smooth sailing and a rocky marriage or partnership.

Gina and Trent's problems with financial stress were typical. Trent's website design business was losing money, and all of a sudden the couple's budget became extremely tight. Gina was frustrated that she couldn't afford to continue her tennis lessons and membership at the gym, where she'd made new friends. One of the hardest things for Trent was that he had to put off buying the new computer and smartphone he'd been eager to buy. The couple soon found themselves arguing over what to spend money on, which took a huge toll on their happiness. Both felt isolated, alone, and scared. They wanted to work things out but didn't know how. Their positive interactions became fewer and farther between, with more time spent disagreeing over money. Would their relationship and marriage succumb to their financial crisis? How could they work things out during this rough period?

Put yourself in Trent or Gina's shoes. Which of the stress management techniques from Part II might be helpful for this couple? How would you suggest Trent and Gina use them? Write in your suggestions in the worksheet on the facing page.

Since their communication was suffering, Trent and Gina turned to the skills in Chapter 6 to help them develop better speaking and listening skills. They also used the material in this chapter on disagreements (page 254) to help them practice more solid communication skills. This enabled both to feel better about sharing their thoughts and feelings about their current financial situation. Gina felt closer to Trent just knowing that he listened and really understood how upset she was about having to give up some of the social activities she used to enjoy. Once the lines of communication were reopened,

---

Should You Have a Joint Bank Account, Separate Accounts, or Both?

Use the communication strategies you learned in Chapter 6 to discuss with your partner or spouse how you want to keep your money. Some prefer to have a joint account and have all expenses taken out of it. Others prefer two separate (and private) accounts and a joint account for household expenses. The stress arises when decisions are made unilaterally or without open, honest, and continuing communication. Resentment can crop up when you least expect it if you start to feel as if the financial burdens aren't shared equitably.

TRENT AND GINA'S FINANCIAL STRESS MANAGEMENT STRATEGIES

Stress management technique	Use
1.	
2.	
3.	
4.	

the couple used the problem-solving techniques from Chapter 5 to help them come up with ways to stretch their thinning budget. Together they began keeping closer track of their monthly income and expenses, which helped them see eye to eye on things. They used their communication skills to hear each other out and make decisions about which expenses to cut and which to keep. An idea that appealed to them, and which helped them feel like a couple again, was to plan "in-home" date nights involving renting a movie and preparing a home-cooked meal to eat by candlelight. If your relationship is affected by financial stressors, it might be helpful to also find a financial advisor who can analyze your particular situation and make suggestions about where to cut and whether it's a good idea to make any investments.

THE HOLIDAYS

You're supposed to be festive and full of cheer at the holidays—which is why it's easy to take holiday stress for granted. But the fact is you probably have higher expectations for this season than for any other time of the year. And all of the planning and stressing at holiday time can leave you feeling cranky, overwhelmed, impatient, anxious, and even depressed.

Holiday Stress

Holiday time becomes stressful when your expectations clash with reality. You want to enjoy every minute, give (and receive) the perfect gifts, and host a flawless celebration with just the right festive atmosphere. Everyone in the family should be together, get along, agree with your ideas for how to celebrate, and so on.

So, if you get stressed during the holidays, examining your expectations is a good place to start. It will help you pinpoint potential stressors and stressful cognitions. In the worksheet at the bottom of this page, write down what you expect from yourself and from family and friends at holiday time.

The next step is to look at whether your expectations fall into any of the categories of stress-inducing cognitions from Chapter 8. Are there any signs of *must*urbation (are your expectations actually *demands*)? Do you notice any all-or-nothing thinking (can you not enjoy the holidays unless *everything's* perfect)? Maybe there are signs of awfulizing (would it be *terrible* if the family wasn't all together?). Perhaps your expectations are simply unrealistic (such as getting the entire family together in one place).

If some of your expectations are unrealistic or contain stress-provoking cognitions, you're certainly not alone. But the best form of stress management for these sorts of cognitions is cognitive therapy. Can you turn your *must*urbatory demands into personal preferences or wishes? Can you convince yourself that although there might be disappointments during the holidays, it's probably not truly *awful* (and remember, the holiday season is over before you know it). Use the worksheet on the facing page to write down your stress-provoking cognitions about the holidays, ways to challenge these beliefs, and the stress-reducing alternative cognitions. Aim for realistic beliefs and attitudes about

HOLIDAY EXPECTATIONS

I expect myself to:	I expect my family (and friends) to:

your goals for the holidays and your expectations of the other people in your life. I've included an example to get you started.

Holiday Blues

The holidays were stressful for Leena, but in a different way. She found herself feeling sad, lonely, and angry, especially when she saw everyone else so full of cheer. Leena and her husband had just separated, and she was thinking stressful thoughts like "I'm such a loser for not having anyone to celebrate the holidays with," "Everyone else is happy and in love except me," and "This is going to be awful." Leena felt empty inside—like she wanted to go to sleep before Thanksgiving and not wake up until sometime in the middle of January. And since things at work tended to slow down as the holidays drew near, she had lots of time to stew about how terrible her situation would be.

REPLACING STRESS-PROVOKING THOUGHTS ABOUT THE HOLIDAYS

Stress-*provoking* cognition	Challenges	Stress-*reducing* cognition
Aunt Carol should come on time this year so we can all open presents together.	*Can I control what Carol does and whether she's late? Will people understand if we open presents without her? It's a nice idea, but is it true that we absolutely <u>must</u> all be together to open presents?*	*Carol is her own person, and I can't make her be on time. The rest of the family knows she has a problem with lateness and will understand if we start without her. I'd prefer for us all to open gifts as a happy family, but if not, it's hardly the end of the world!*

If holiday time is marked by feeling down and depressed (rather than anxious or worried about things going just right), then, like Leena, you might have what's known as the "holiday blues." Here are some of the factors that can contribute to feeling blue at holiday time:

- You associate the holidays with unsettling or painful childhood or family issues.

- You've recently lost a loved one with whom you're used to sharing the holidays.

- You're spending the holidays away from family and friends, or feel isolated.

- You're coping with a relationship breakup or divorce.

But even under these circumstances, you can use the techniques from Part II to reduce your stress at holiday time. Given Leena's overly negative thinking patterns, hopefully you'd agree that cognitive therapy is a good place for her to start. What kinds of stress-reducing thoughts can you come up with that might help her lessen her stress and depression? Write them in the following spaces.

_____

_____

_____

_____

Revamping her thinking patterns helped Leena accept that, at least for this year, the holiday season would be a challenge. But at least it's a relatively short period of time—she would get through it. She tried to stop *expecting* to feel good just because it was the holidays. Below I list some other strategies that can help you manage stress if you're feeling blue at holiday time. Think about which ones might be helpful for you.

- Take a vacation to someplace nice during the holidays (alone or with a relative or friend) to change your routine so you're not feeling like you're sitting around and missing out.

- Spend time with people who care about you.

- Reduce your feelings of isolation by volunteering and helping others.

- Get yourself wrapped up in working on a project or learning a new skill or hobby.

- Hit the gym, work on your physical fitness, and learn some new exercises. Set realistic short-term goals for what you want to accomplish before the holidays are over.

- Use meditation to clear your mind of distressing thoughts and emotions and allow yourself to enjoy whatever pleasant moments occur in the here and now.

DEALING WITH A DIFFICULT RELATIVE

Is there someone in your family who acts obnoxiously, insensitively, intrusively, or who grates on your nerves in other ways? Maybe you have to deal with this person only at family gatherings once in a while. Okay, you can put up with anyone for a few hours at a time. But maybe it's worse than that. Maybe you have to interact with this relative on a regular basis—or even deal with him or her routinely when it comes to handling various family issues.

Barbara and Kim were sisters, each with her own family of grown-up children. But Barbara found dealing with her sister maddening. After a phone call, e-mail, or in-person interaction, she'd usually find herself distracted and impatient. She'd have trouble concentrating at work, trying to relax, or trying to get to sleep. And she'd walk around the house angry, tense, and irritable—like she just wanted to scream! It was like the two were never on the same page about anything, and years of experience told Barbara that it was useless trying to communicate rationally with Kim. While Barbara was poised, confident, sensible, and generous with others, Kim seemed reckless and impulsive, insecure, self-centered, and even spiteful.

Take the situation with their mother, who was a widow and becoming more and more isolated and less able to live on her own. Barbara wanted her to move to a senior adult living community, which would provide a more supportive and stimulating environment and round-the-clock medical care if needed. Kim, on the other hand, didn't want to sell the home where she'd grown up. And *she* wanted to be the one her mother depended on for support, stimulation, and care now that Dad was gone (even though she'd proven unreliable in providing such care). So Kim tried to sabotage Barbara's plans to move their mother by spreading nasty rumors about the senior living community to other members of their family in hopes of turning them against Barbara. While Barbara wanted what was best for their mother, Kim was trying to undermine this for her own personal reasons. And she wouldn't even listen to Barbara when she tried to explain the many reasons their mother belonged in the senior community.

To get some relief from her stress, Barbara turned to cognitive therapy (Chapter 8) to help modify stressful thinking patterns. But she found this only somewhat helpful. She'd long ago lowered her expectations of Kim's behavior. And although she had lots of negative thoughts about Kim, focusing them on her behavior (rather than labeling her sister as a bad or incompetent *person*) didn't relieve much stress. That's when Barbara turned to problem solving. But rather than trying to work things out with Kim— Barbara felt it would only increase stress to try to find common ground with her sister— she got creative and came up with the following strategies for managing stress related to her sister. If you have a relative who triggers stress in a similar way, think about how you can apply these strategies.

Build Stronger Alliances with Family Members You Do Enjoy

Barbara had solid relationships with her cousins, who were sensitive and caring and knew about Kim's behavior. So she set aside time each month to get together with them for lunch or an evening out. Although sometimes these turned into gossip sessions, Barbara did her best to steer the conversations toward other, less stressful, topics. Who are some family members you can connect with for support in dealing with your difficult relative?

_____

_____

Remind Yourself of Reasons Not to Give Up Trying to Deal with the Person

Maybe your difficult relative is married or close to someone in your family that you do enjoy and don't want to see get hurt. Barbara had nothing against Kim's husband and two sons (each married with families of their own). In fact, she felt a certain bond with them since they all had to put up with Kim's behavior. Barbara also tried to remind herself that dealing with Kim was an opportunity to learn important lessons about patience, persistence, and setting limits. Think about your own reasons for not giving up and write them in the following spaces.

_____

_____

_____

Maybe you just believe that blood is thicker than water and it's important to try to work things out with family members. Perhaps you recognize that you and this other person both have a stubborn side and that it's possible for each of you to give some ground to come to an agreement. You don't have to discuss your reasons with anyone, but keep them in mind so that the effort you make to deal with your difficult relative will feel worthwhile.

Set Small, Achievable Goals for "Successful" Interactions

Years of dealing with Kim had lowered Barbara's expectations for interactions with her sister. She knew that most of them would go nowhere. So she started trying to think of ways to feel successful about her inevitable interactions with Kim. She set small and realistic goals, such as keeping phone calls civil and no longer than 10 minutes. If your relative has a habit of giving you too much advice, you could set a goal such as listening to one piece of advice and saying "That's interesting; I'll consider it" without getting into a debate. If your difficult relative likes to talk about other relatives behind their backs, you could set the goal of speaking up and asking that the conversation not involve putting others down. When it comes to difficult family members, remind yourself that you don't need to change this person's basic personality—what's important is staying healthy, calm, and relaxed no matter what he or she does. What realistic goals can you set?

_____

_____

_____

Look for New Ways to Connect

As adults, there weren't too many times when Barbara and Kim saw eye to eye. But growing up in the same family, Barbara knew the activities, places, and topics that she and her sister both enjoyed. So she tried to bring out the best in Kim by bringing up these topics and suggesting these activities, rather than repeating the same old interactions that hadn't worked for years. What are ways that you could connect positively and peacefully with your difficult relative? Is there a show or movie you both enjoy? Or an art museum, sporting or musical event, or old family photo album? Be proactive and from time to time schedule a brief activity that has a high likelihood of bringing out the best in both of you. List the possible topics and activities you could suggest:

_____

_____

_____

13

Managing a Crisis

A *crisis* is an unexpected and overwhelming event that creates major changes in your life and, therefore, intense stress. You might have to make important decisions and take action in the wake of a crisis, either to minimize damage or to adapt to life changes thrust upon you. Some crisis situations, such as medical emergencies, assaults, and natural disasters, involve actual (or threatened) injury, harm, or danger. Others involve devastating loss, such as having your home burglarized, unexpectedly losing a loved one, and (sometimes) losing your job. Whatever the event, the most important defining factor with respect to stress is that a crisis carries with it the prospect of changes so significant to your life that your ability to cope may be stretched to its limit.

Much of what you've learned in this book so far is aimed at preventing everyday stress from mushrooming out of control. The tools and techniques presented in earlier chapters will serve you well in a crisis situation too, but some additional measures can help you prevent the stress of a crisis from doing long-term damage. There are also some types of help that are often more critical in a crisis, such as support from family and friends, than they would be with everyday stress. It's particularly important not to feel

In a true crisis you experience physical and emotional harm or loss, and your ability to cope is stretched to the limit.

alone during a crisis, and that means not only enlisting the support of others but also understanding that your responses are normal and universal. This chapter will help you use the techniques learned in Part II of this workbook to get through what's probably a very difficult and stressful period of time.

COMMON RESPONSES TO A CRISIS: FEELING SHOCKED AND OVERWHELMED

Marta returned from work to find her front door wide open. From standing outside, she could see that her possessions had been strewn all over the place. Heart pounding, she ran back to her car and called the police. When officers arrived and eventually said it was safe to go inside, Marta was totally unprepared for what she saw. Clothes had been tossed everywhere, furniture knocked over, dresser drawers had been emptied, and jewelry and other valuables were gone. Her television, stereo, DVD collection, artwork, and laptop computer had been taken, along with some of her clothes, shoes, and the holiday gifts she had just shopped for. Marta's first response was a mix of anger ("How could someone do this!?") and worry ("What if they come back to hurt me?"). As she walked through her home answering questions from the police officers, the recurring thoughts of an intruder going through all of her personal belongings made Marta feel extremely violated and unsafe. She was shaken. What would she do next?

Jonas was driving Tara home from their date when another car crossed the center lane and caused a head-on collision. Jonas was disoriented after the crash, but he wasn't seriously hurt. Tara, on the other hand, was gravely injured. She was taken to the hospital, but the doctors couldn't save her life. When Jonas became aware of what had happened, he was in a state of shock. For weeks, he could think of nothing but the accident and what had happened to Tara. He felt shaky and jittery all the time, had trouble sleeping, and even had recurring nightmares about the accident. He was filled with grief and guilt. "I'm responsible for Tara's death. It's all my fault," he told himself. Jonas avoided getting back on the road for fear of having another accident. He just wanted to stay at home and be alone in his room—which is how he spent the next few weeks. Nothing seemed to matter. Would things ever return to normal?

Virginia's son, Ezra, was only five years old when he came down with pneumonia—a very serious lung infection. It started with what seemed like a bad cold, but soon progressed to fevers, chest pain, and trouble breathing. After 6 weeks in the hospital, Ezra's lungs became so weak that he died. Even though the doctors had told Virginia a few weeks earlier to prepare for the worst—which Virginia had tried to do—Ezra's death still sent her into a state of shock. Initially, she was in denial: how could this all have happened so fast? Then she became grief stricken. She had recurring nightmares and flashbacks—images of little Ezra's lifeless body. She isolated herself from everyone, even her family, who was trying to give her support. Virginia lost weight because of her depression and guilt and had trouble sleeping. She even started blaming herself for not taking Ezra to the doctor sooner. He was her only child—how could she go on?

Everyone responds a little differently to a crisis. But as the preceding examples show, the most common response is *mental shock*—an intense form of stress that involves disbelief, numbness, confusion, and a feeling of disconnection. You might have trouble thinking about anything else but the crisis. You might feel unsafe or unable to trust others. You might have trouble sleeping, eating, or socializing. Your degree of mental shock, and how long it lasts, will depend on things such as the seriousness of the crisis, your involvement, the degree of threat to life and limb, how life-changing it is, and other factors. But it's important to understand that some level of mental shock in the wake of a crisis is normal. In fact, mental shock is your mind and body's way of dealing with crisis or psychological trauma. That is, almost everyone who goes through a crisis experiences it in one way or another. Fortunately, for most people, psychological shock is short-lived. It might last several days or weeks, but then it gradually lifts most of the time . . . though not always.

Look at the list of mental shock symptoms in the worksheet below. Do you experience any of these? Using the scale from 0 to 4, rate the intensity of each of these problems in the wake of your crisis situation.

What symptoms have you been experiencing? How intense are they? You might have noticed that some of the symptoms are connected to others. For example, feeling guilty might lead to despair and depression, and flashbacks or nightmares might make you feel out of control, leading to anxiety, fear, and increased physical arousal. It's easy to become scared and overwhelmed by mental shock. Some people worry that these

INTENSITY OF SHOCK SYMPTOMS FOLLOWING A CRISIS

Describe the crisis situation: _____

How many days, weeks, or months ago did the crisis occur? _____

Rating scale

0 = none   1 = mild   2 = moderate   3 = severe   4 = extreme

Shock symptoms	Rating (circle)
Fear and anxiety that last long after the crisis situation is over	0 1 2 3 4
Reexperiencing the crisis situation through unwanted thoughts, nightmares, flashbacks, or vivid images as if the crisis were occurring again	0 1 2 3 4
Increased physical arousal, including feeling jumpy, jittery, shaky, being easily startled, trouble concentrating, and difficulty sleeping	0 1 2 3 4
Impatience, anger, and irritability or the feeling that the world is not fair or is a dangerous and unpredictable place	0 1 2 3 4
Avoidance of situations or people that remind you of the crisis situation	0 1 2 3 4
Guilt and shame and blaming yourself (or taking responsibility) for the crisis even if it's not actually your fault	0 1 2 3 4
Depression and feelings of sadness, hopelessness, shame, helplessness, worthlessness, confusion, despair; crying; losing interest in people or activities you used to enjoy	0 1 2 3 4
Lowered self-esteem	0 1 2 3 4
Reduced trust in other people	0 1 2 3 4
Trouble feeling sexual or having sexual relationships	0 1 2 3 4

symptoms mean they're losing control or going crazy. But it's important to remember that this is a normal process that's part of your body's fight-or-flight system. You will not lose control or "go crazy" from the shock symptoms.

How long ago did your crisis situation occur? As I mentioned before, for most people, the initial symptoms of mental shock wear off on their own as time passes—although this can take from a day or two to a month or more. If your crisis occurred within the last 3 months, it's very likely that your shock symptoms will lessen even if you don't do anything about them. But if it's been more than 3 months since your crisis, and you've rated some of the symptoms on page 272 as 3 (severe) or 4 (extreme), you might be struggling with posttraumatic stress disorder, or PTSD. PTSD is a serious (and treatable) psychological disorder in which the symptoms of mental shock become more or less permanent and require professional help to get over. If you're experiencing the symptoms that Johanna had (described in the box below), it's probably worth seeking

---

Johanna's Signs and Symptoms of PTSD

One evening, walking to her car in the parking lot of a local shopping center, Johanna was attacked. A tall man wearing a ski mask grabbed her from behind, flashed a gun, and demanded that she give him her purse and car keys. The man pushed Johanna to the ground, yelled at her, and then fled in her car. Johanna wasn't badly hurt, but she was in shock. She experienced the typical symptoms of PTSD as follows:

Johanna began having unwanted memories, flashbacks, and nightmares of the mugging—as if playing a movie of it in her head over and over—and she couldn't stop these from coming up. She also started avoiding any reminders of the terrible event, such as the mall where it happened. She didn't even want her car returned. When something did remind her, she suddenly felt extremely upset and uncomfortable; her heart would start thumping loudly in her chest, she'd feel like she couldn't catch her breath, and she'd clench her muscles, particularly in her jaw and neck, leading to muscle soreness after the episode had ended.

These episodes were even more upsetting and bewildering to Johanna because she couldn't recall everything that had happened during the mugging: How could she keep replaying the attack when her memory of it was so spotty? Meanwhile, she couldn't sleep, she found herself losing her temper in situations that would have rolled off her back in the past, and she was constantly looking over her shoulder, jumping at the slightest sound behind her and so distracted by arming herself mentally for the next attack that her concentration was suffering at work. What was worse, however, was that she started to feel emotionless, as if she just didn't care—not only about the job she used to love but also about her friends, her family, and the pursuits she used to be passionate about. Maybe it didn't matter, she told herself. After all, she wasn't sure how long she would live. Sometimes she had the sense that her life would be cut short even though she had escaped the mugger. And there was also self-blame: "If I had fought back, this never would have happened," she told herself. When these thoughts started to keep her up at night, she turned to alcohol—first just to get to sleep and then to ease her aching muscles after dinner. Johanna was vaguely aware that she was sinking into depression and often felt lonely and hopeless, but she had no idea what to do about it.

an evaluation from a qualified mental health professional. Remember, it's not a sign of weakness to get help when you need it; rather, it's a smart and responsible way to take care of yourself.

First Steps: Coping Immediately after a Crisis

Even if you don't have full-fledged mental shock symptoms, you're likely to feel very overwhelmed when you face a crisis. Regardless, practicing stress management skills in the aftermath of a crisis could mean the difference between a healthy recovery and developing longer-term problems such as PTSD or depression. Here are some suggestions for how to cope in the immediate aftermath of a crisis.

Concentrate on What's Most Important

Depending on the nature of the crisis, you may not have any choice but to spend all your time and energy on dealing with its repercussions. Nevertheless, you might feel like you need to meet your usual daily responsibilities too. While the extra mental, emotional, and physical exertion can obviously increase your stress, meeting your other normal obligations may relieve the stress of worrying about falling behind on work or personal tasks. This is where taking a break to practice mindfulness, do some progressive relaxation, lie down for a few minutes, or take a brisk walk—whatever you have learned helps you clear your mind—can be a lifesaver. As you relieve a little of the pressure of the moment, you may find yourself better able to use problem-solving tools to determine what's best for you and your stress level: Forget about the everyday responsibilities for now and concentrate on managing the crisis itself? Keep busy, staying on top of your daily tasks? You might find that a balance is best, meaning that instead of simply ignoring the daily necessities, you find someone to help.

Right after a crisis, just getting through the day might seem like a major accomplishment. You need all the physical and mental energy you can muster. So, prioritize what's necessary to help you cope and allow yourself to put other duties and responsibilities on the back burner if meeting them will cause you more stress than putting them aside for a while—other people will understand. For example, can you excuse yourself from PTA meetings, let others help you with shopping and cooking if they volunteer to do so, and think about taking a few days off from work or school? Read page 137 in Chapter 7 on getting organized and making a to-do list. What are some ways you can cut back to conserve your energy? Jot them down on the following lines.

_____

_____

_____

_____

Get Social Support

If you let others know about your crisis, chances are they'll offer to help you, *and this is the time to take them up on it*. Let loved ones lighten your load by helping with tasks or just providing a supportive ear (you'll repay their favors later, when you're up to it). Getting social support will build your morale and help you feel better. Whom can you turn to for support? Enter their names in the following spaces.

_____

_____

Stay Healthy

When you're drained of physical and mental energy, the last thing you need is to let good eating, sleeping, and exercise habits slip by the wayside. But it's easy to forgo these in times of crisis because your normal routine is turned upside down. Think about ways you can stay healthy (such as asking people not to bring you a pan of brownies to help out, but a homemade soup or pasta; and going on walks while talking to people who can give you support—refer to Chapter 10 for more pointers) and write them in the following blanks:

_____

_____

_____

_____

Sort Out Your Thoughts and Feelings

A crisis can be so shattering and so different from your everyday experiences that you don't know how to make sense of it. Remember Marta? She'd never imagined feeling so unsafe in her own home. And Jonas never expected his date with Tara to end so tragically. After a crisis, your mind keeps bringing up thoughts and memories of the event (sometimes as intrusive thoughts, images, nightmares, and flashbacks) as if to digest the trauma and integrate it with what you know about the world. While you might be tempted to try to ignore or push away these unpleasant thoughts and feelings, allowing your mind to process and think them through is actually the way to get a better grasp and eventually let them go. Putting words to your experience—using a journal, talking to a loved one, or consulting a therapist—can be an important step. Meditation is another. What are some ways you can help your mind digest the crisis you've been through?

_____

_____

Be Patient

Remember that the mental shock reactions you read about on pages 270–273 are entirely normal after experiencing a crisis. Accept them and accept yourself. Take time to relax (using the techniques in Chapter 10, for example) and reflect in ways that are comfortable for you. Often it's a matter of time before things settle back down.

The next part of this chapter will help you manage stress associated with particular types of crises. You'll get the most out of these sections if you use the techniques once the initial shock of your crisis has begun to dissipate (or is less intense), allowing you to focus more clearly.

HOUSEHOLD CRISES: BURGLARIES AND FIRES

Your home—whether a house, apartment, or otherwise—is your sanctuary. Think about the time, energy, and money you've put into making it a comfortable place where you can feel safe. When you're at home, you're surrounded by familiar things. Maybe you have lots of sentimental belongings—pictures, books, family heirlooms, and the like. Your home is an extension of yourself. That's why having it destroyed by fire or flood, or ravaged by an intruder, is an extremely traumatic experience that leaves you feeling shocked, disoriented, unsafe, and violated. Consider what happened to Ron's family:

If you've lost a loved one in a crisis, refer to pages 288–289 later in this chapter for help with managing your thoughts and emotions.

Ron was out of town on business when he received the dreadful phone call from his wife. A heater with faulty wiring had set fire to a wall in Ron's home office, which destroyed their home, killing the family pets, and throwing everything into chaos. Ron hopped on the next flight home and arrived to see burning ashes and a safe yet disoriented family. Normally very poised and self-confident, Ron found himself unable to think straight. He was stunned and didn't seem to know what to do. He was grateful that his family was alive, but they'd lost everything. They didn't even have a place to sit down and come up with a plan for moving forward.

If you're reading this chapter after suffering a crisis in your home—such as a fire, burglary, storm damage, or other catastrophe—here are some ways to get the most out of the stress management techniques taught in Part II of this workbook once you've taken care of the practical necessities.

Breaking Down the Stressors

You feel small and powerless after a household crisis. And you're overwhelmed with so much to do. This is where the problem-solving techniques described in Chapter 5 can come in handy. Think about it this way: how would you approach other large projects such as planning a wedding, starting a business, or buying a new car? You'd start by breaking down the big task into smaller, more manageable chunks. Maybe you already know what problems need to be solved in the wake of your crisis. If not, use the Recognizing Problems section in Chapter 5 (Step 1) to help you identify any you've missed or that are still triggering stress. Once you have your problem list, you'll

> *When you're in crisis mode, it's easy to forget that the same organizational skills you use every day can also carry you through difficult times.*

need to prioritize them according to urgency and other factors, such as how much help you need and when or where you can get the help. Chapter 7 on time management can help you with these decisions. For example, you might make a list of problems you can solve on your own versus those that require assistance. Don't be afraid to ask others to help you out when you need it.

Thinking Straight

Dealing with Lost or Damaged Property

Even with effective problem solving, once your home has been damaged, destroyed, or burglarized, you'll probably face stress-provoking questions such as "Will I ever get my stolen items back? Can the parts of my home that were damaged be completely fixed? How can I replace sentimental or one-of-a-kind items that were lost?" If you're lucky, some of what was stolen, lost, or damaged can be recovered or restored. But not always; and if there are important or sentimental things that you can't replace, fix, or recover,

> *Don't use cognitive therapy to try to talk yourself into feeling happy at a time like this. You've got to be honest and acknowledge the loss, hurt, and feelings of violation. But at the same time, if you're realistic, you're in a better frame of mind to deal with the practical side of managing your crisis.*

adjusting to this fact can be a very stressful experience. As with other situations that you can't manipulate directly, the best way to manage your stress here will be to use cognitive therapy to identify and challenge the thinking patterns that create stress over these unfortunate circumstances. Common stressful beliefs include "I can't stand not having _____" and "How can I go on without _____?" Can you identify your own? Write them in the worksheet on the next page. Then use the techniques taught in Chapter 8

to help you come up with healthier, stress-reducing thoughts to use going forward. These should acknowledge the hurt of being victimized, but also the opportunities that the crisis has opened up. For example, "I hate that the burglar stole my guitar, but that gives me

---

THINKING STRAIGHT ABOUT PROPERTY LOSS OR DAMAGE

My stress-provoking thoughts about loss:

My stress-reducing thoughts:

---

an excuse to buy the better one that I was checking out" or "The fire was pretty bad, but we'll survive. I guess we have an opportunity to redecorate the house as we'd like."

Dealing with Self-Blame

Are you blaming yourself and feeling guilty about causing your crisis? This is a common—but stress-provoking—response. Ron's wife, for example, believed she was at fault for her family's house fire and subsequent losses since she happened to be the one who'd left the faulty heater on in Ron's home office. But was the fire really her fault? After all, accidents happen—and it wasn't like she knew the heater was defective. If you're blaming yourself, you'll need to work on changing your thinking and chalking the crisis up to a very unfortunate or unpredictable event. This will also help you reduce your stress. Use the worksheet on the facing page, and the techniques in Chapter 8, to assist you.

Dealing with Feeling Unsafe

Do you feel insecure and unsafe—even in your own home? These feelings are normal after a crisis such as a severe fire or burglary, but they still come from thinking patterns like jumping to conclusions (for example, "It happened once, so it's bound to happen again"). Fortunately, these stressful thoughts and feelings often dissipate by themselves as time goes by and you realize that your crisis is not likely to be repeated. You can help

THINKING STRAIGHT ABOUT FEELING GUILTY

My stress-provoking thoughts about guilt:

My stress-reducing thoughts:

this process along using cognitive therapy to challenge exaggerated estimates of the probability of fires and burglaries (for example, using questions such as "What are the actual odds of these events occurring?" and "Could the fact that I was just robbed be influencing how likely I think it is to happen again?"). Use the Thinking Straight about Danger and Safety worksheet (page 280) to help you.

If you're still feeling very unsafe, on edge, insecure, or worried about a repeat of the crisis after several weeks of practicing cognitive therapy, it's time to look at what might be getting in the way of changing your cognitions. Ironically, you might be relying on certain "coping strategies" that, when used to excess, backfire and make you even more stressed. Read the list of strategies that follows and put a check next to any that you've started doing since your crisis:

❒ Avoiding staying at home alone or at night

❒ Avoiding using electrical appliances such as the oven, stove, or iron

❒ Avoiding lighting matches, candles, or a fire in the fireplace

❒ Installing extra (more than one) deadbolt locks (including on a bedroom door)

❒ Installing extra (more than one) security or fire alarm systems

❒ Installing extra fire extinguishers

THINKING STRAIGHT ABOUT DANGER AND SAFETY

My stress-provoking thoughts about danger and safety:

My stress-reducing thought about danger and safety:

❏ Installing a camera to monitor activity outside your house

❏ Buying a weapon

❏ Checking and rechecking locks, windows, appliances, outlets, the fire or burglar alarm system, and the like

❏ Checking with others for assurance (that is, asking them lots of questions about safety in the home)

So, you *do* use some of these strategies? It's understandable—after all, they seem to make perfect sense. First, they might make you feel more comfortable. Second, nothing terrible has happened since you started using them, right? But these kinds of strategies can have negative side effects. That's because they rob you of opportunities to realize that you're actually much safer than you think and that this crisis is extremely unlikely to repeat itself even if you didn't use these strategies. In other words, these kinds of strategies can *increase* your stress.

Let's take avoidance. When you stay away from home, avoid being alone at night, or refuse to use appliances or fire in safe ways (such as using candles or a gas stove), you never have the chance to see that these situations are actually safer than you've been thinking. Avoidance also prevents you from learning to feel comfortable in these situations again. As a result, you continue to feel that they're very dangerous and that you'd go on being anxious forever if you didn't avoid them.

It's basically the same with excessive checking, installing extra safety measures, and asking for assurances: all of these strategies might make you feel like you're protecting yourself, but if there's very little risk to begin with, what good do they do? They only reinforce your thoughts that your home is a dangerous place, that disaster is likely, and that you've always got to be on guard to prevent a crisis. Sleeping with a gun under your pillow, for example, is only going to remind you of how much you expect an intruder to burst in at any moment—even though it's very unlikely to actually happen.

How can you prove this to yourself and start feeling safe again in your own home? It turns out that this requires finding ways to eliminate these "coping strategies" so you can see what really happens. And that's not an easy task if you're stressed about another crisis. So, let me help you through this process.

Begin by flipping back to the checklist on pages 279–280. Which strategies do you rely on to make you feel safer than you already are? In the first column of the Stopping Unhelpful Coping Strategies worksheet on page 282, list these, and any other specific situations you avoid, as well as any other precautions you take to prevent or protect you from another crisis. Examples might include avoiding using the oven, sleeping with a weapon under the bed, installing extra locks on the front door (or a bedroom door), and avoiding lighting matches.

There's no need to stop all of these strategies at once. In fact, an approach that works for most people is to figure out which are easier to eliminate and work on those first, before moving on to more difficult ones. That's why I've included the column marked "order" in the worksheet. Think about which strategies would be easy, moderate, and difficult to stop and put a number in this column that corresponds to the order in which you'll work on ending each one.

The next step is to plan *how* you'll eliminate each unhelpful coping strategy (and write your plan in the appropriate column in the worksheet). There are a number of ways you can try eliminating these strategies. Here are some suggestions:

- For situations you avoid, such as staying at home alone at night, try easing yourself into it. For example, start by staying at home alone during the day. Then try it at night, but arrange for a friend or relative to check up on you (either by phone or in person). Then try it with no check-ins. Think of how great you'll feel the next morning when you've reclaimed your space.

- If you avoid *activities* such as using the oven or lighting a match, a similar tactic can help: First, try doing the activity with someone else (or a fire extinguisher) nearby "just in case." But gradually remove these safety cues until it's just *you* doing the activity alone. You'll find that your estimations of the danger level decrease when you master these activities again.

- If you've turned your home into a maximum-security fortress because of your fear that intruders will return, try gradually reducing the use of cameras, extra locks, and security systems. Of course, keep all doors and windows locked (a general safety precaution for anyone)—but don't lock any inside doors, and you need only a single

STOPPING UNHELPFUL COPING STRATEGIES

	Strategy	Order	Elimination plan	Completed
1.				
2.				
3.				
4.				
5.				
6.				
7.				
8.				
9.				
10.				

deadbolt lock on any door to the outside. If you have a built-in security system, then by all means use it. But don't use extra measures such as exterior cameras.

- If you've bought extra weapons, or are keeping weapons with you when you sleep (such as a gun under your bed), start by putting them somewhere else in your room for the night. Then move them to an adjacent room, and so on, until you feel more comfortable being home (and sleeping) with them locked away in a safe place. It might take some time, but you'll find that when you keep your weapons in their rightful place (rather than always within reach), you'll become less and less sensitive (and less reactive) to every little noise you hear at night. And you'll think less about intruders.

- If you've developed the habit of checking and rechecking, try gradually cutting down the number of times you check or the different places you check.

Managing High Anxiety during Anti-Stress Experiments

Be prepared: when you begin your anti-stress experiments, it's likely that you'll provoke anxiety or fear. It might feel like you're walking a tightrope and someone has taken away your safety net! But don't give in when your discomfort increases; these anxious feelings are temporary. They'll subside on their own when you give them a chance. In the meantime, remind yourself that these feelings are temporary and harmless—and you can cope with them. More important, when you let these feelings come down on their own, you'll start to feel that you don't need these "coping" strategies because you're a much better tightrope walker than you'd thought!

Instead of stressing yourself out further by telling yourself how terrible it feels to let go of the coping strategies, try repeating to yourself the stress-reducing cognitions from page 280. You can also use these coping statements to help you ride out the temporary feelings of stress and anxiety:

- "Anxiety is normal and temporary. Think how good it will feel when it subsides."

- "The anxious sensations feel *uncomfortable*, but they're not *dangerous*."

- "I have to make myself anxious to get better."

- "If I stop now, I'll only be making my stress worse."

- "It's worth deciding to be anxious in the short run to get over this problem in the long run."

- "I can handle this. I can let the anxiety decrease by itself—no matter how long it takes."

Don't try to use these coping statements to make your anxiety go away. Rather, let them inspire you to *ride it out*. You don't have to *enjoy* being anxious, but it's a part of life that you've got to accept if you're going to reduce the impact of stress on your life.

Once you've got a plan for eliminating each unhelpful coping strategy, you're ready to start. Each time you implement part of your plan, we'll treat it as an experiment (an "anti-stress" experiment) in which you're testing out (or "putting on trial") your beliefs about danger, safety, or the risks of another crisis. Take a look at the Anti-Stress Experiment worksheet below. Each time you work toward reducing or eliminating a unhelpful coping strategy, complete the form (make copies for multiple use) so you can learn from your experiences.

Start by describing the experiment you're doing, such as "leaving the kitchen for 10 minutes while I'm cooking food in the oven." Next, write out your "stress forecast," which is similar to a weather forecast—a prediction about what you think will happen. In this case, it's the *worst possible* prediction; such as "The oven will catch fire and the house will burn down." The next step is to rate the likelihood (from 0 to 100%) that your stress forecast is accurate. What are the chances it will happen? Finally, before you start, rate your stress level on a scale from 0 (not at all stressed) to 100 (*extremely* stressed out). Then test out your stress forecast by conducting your experiment.

When you've finished the experiment (or the next day, if your experiment runs overnight), again rate your stress level. Then describe the outcome of your experiment.

ANTI-STRESS EXPERIMENT

1. Describe the experiment: _____

_____

2. Specific stress forecast (describe): _____

_____

3. What are the chances (likelihood) of your stress forecast being correct (0–100%)? _____

4. Stress level immediately before beginning the experiment (0–100%) _____

5. Stress level immediately after completing the experiment (0–100%) _____

6. Describe the outcome of the experiment. What happened (or *didn't* happen)? _____

_____

_____

7. What is the revised chance that the stress forecast is correct (0–100%)? _____

8. Based on this experience, what crisis experiment should I try next? _____

_____

What happened? Was your stress forecast correct or not? How did you feel afterward? After writing down a revised likelihood estimate for your stress forecast (hopefully, your estimate will get lower), consider how the results of this experiment can inform more experiments that can prove to yourself that your threat forecasts are not at all likely. Using cognitive therapy together with reducing your reliance on unhelpful "safety behaviors" (by using anti-stress experiments) will teach you how to feel safe in your own home again.

HEALTH-RELATED CRISES

When a serious health crisis befalls you or a close relative, your life changes quickly. You're diagnosed with a life-threatening medical condition. A loved one is seriously injured or disabled. A relative dies suddenly or prematurely. All of these produce feelings of loss, grief, anxiety, and depression. You might have trouble sleeping or suffer crying spells, lose your appetite, and find yourself wanting to be left alone. Your routine also changes, which produces a great deal of stress. In most instances, people eventually come to terms with these situations; they make adjustments and their stressful emotions and behaviors subside. But if you're still having such stressful feelings and behaviors long after the crisis has hit (say six months or a year or more), it might mean you need to do more to manage your stress. In this section, you'll learn how to apply the various stress management techniques to personal and family health crises.

Receiving a Serious Medical Diagnosis

There is no right or wrong way to cope with being diagnosed with a serious, life-changing, or life-threatening disease (such as cancer)—just coping mechanisms that are more or less helpful. The most helpful strategies are those that reduce your stress by helping you adjust to the situation. While everyone copes a little differently, there are two types of coping strategies, attention and distraction:

- *Attention coping* involves trying to regain control over the situation. Actively learning about the disease you have, and the types of treatments for it, is an example of this sort of strategy. Learning can help you feel less helpless and therefore less stressed.

- *Distraction coping*, on the other hand, reduces your stress by helping you divert your attention away from your health. For example, you throw yourself into an activity or new book. In times of high stress, distraction can keep your emotions from becoming overwhelming.

Although you might use both attention and distraction, you probably prefer one approach over the other, depending on the situation. Let's say you're in a traffic jam—a normally stress-provoking situation. An example of an attention coping strategy would be using your GPS to find another route to your destination. But what if that isn't an option (you're stuck on a highway or don't have a GPS)? You might then use distraction, such as turning on the radio and listening to music or a talk show. These two coping strategies can both be used effectively, alone or together. Here are some examples of each as told to me by people facing serious medical illnesses. You might consider using these to help you manage your own health-related stress. Try to think of other attention or distraction coping strategies that have worked for you in the past and write them in the blank spaces. Don't assume that something you've used to get through a less severe trial won't work for a serious crisis. Every little bit helps.

Attention Coping Strategies

- Gather information about your diagnosis.

- Research treatment options.

- Talk to other people with the same diagnosis about their experiences.

- Begin a journal of your experiences.

- Use cognitive therapy techniques (Chapter 8) to identify and challenge stressful thoughts that lead to self-blame, self-criticism, anxiety, and depression.

- _____

- _____

- _____

Distraction Coping Strategies

- Read a new book—an adventure, a mystery, a romance—whatever you enjoy.

- Listen to music you enjoy.

- Play your favorite game.

- Exercise if possible (take a walk, ride a bike, and so on).

- Watch your favorite movies or television shows.

- Spend time on your hobbies.

- Use meditation or relaxation techniques from Chapter 9.

- Pamper yourself with a long bath, shower, or other soothing diversion.

- Go shopping and treat yourself to something you've been looking to buy.

- Spend time with other adults or enjoy yourself playing with children or grand-children.

- _____
- _____
- _____

Serious Injury or Disability

Theresa, an avid biker, was out for a ride one morning when she was hit by a drunk driver. The back and neck injuries she suffered left her paralyzed from the waist down and confined to a wheelchair. Her first reaction was anger—a very natural and perfectly appropriate response. But as the weeks and months went on, these feelings persisted, and she began feeling more and more depressed to boot. She was second-guessing herself: "If only I'd decided not to go riding, things would be different." And she couldn't see herself adjusting or ever being happy again: "My life isn't worth living if I have to spend it in a wheelchair." Theresa had become isolated, anxious about going out in public, and unable to come to terms with her "new normal."

Though it might take many months to adjust to living with a disability, most people make this adjustment over time. Think about which of the stress management strate-

---

EYE OPENER

Believe in Your Ability to Cope

As I've mentioned, reducing your stress can improve your health prognosis. So, when you're feeling overwhelmed, use cognitive therapy techniques to remind yourself that you'll handle this just as you've used coping skills to handle other difficult situations in your life. Here are some suggestions:

Don't deny your feelings about living with a serious medical condition. There will be ups and downs—some good days and some bad ones. Trying to pretend that you're not angry, sad, or fearful is far more stressful than accepting these feelings and sharing them with others. Meditation techniques from Chapter 9 can help you here. So can challenging stressful thinking patterns, such as "I'll never be happy again," "I'm damaged goods," and "I can't cope with this." Use the techniques in Chapter 8 to help you.

Don't blame yourself. It's easy to look for reasons that you developed an illness—for example, blaming skin cancer on not using sunscreen. But beliefs like this are overly simplistic. They're also destructive and stress-provoking because they undermine your ability to adjust to your diagnosis. Use cognitive techniques to challenge these beliefs and remind yourself that the exact causes of most diseases (such as cancer) are complex and largely remain unknown. Many people with lung cancer never smoked; many people who use sunscreen still get skin cancer; and many people with active lifestyles still suffer from heart problems. Don't fall into the trap of believing that you could have completely prevented your illness just by changing some aspect of your behavior. It's not that simple.

gies from Part II Theresa could use to help her accept her disability and begin living life again.

Given that there was nothing Theresa could do about her injuries, she turned first to cognitive therapy. She had a choice: she could be bitter, angry, and depressed over what happened to her, or she could work to accept her situation, look for opportunities to be productive and enjoy things as a person with physical disabilities, and come to view being in a wheelchair as an *inconvenience* that prevented her from enjoying other things (such as biking). To help her along, she took to reading inspiring stories of people who'd achieved great things despite being confined to a wheelchair. These strategies were often effective, but adding meditation really helped her clear her mind of negative thinking. The combination of these techniques, seeking moral support from friends and relatives, and using assertive communication to ask for help (which she wasn't used to doing) helped Theresa reduce her stress and move on with her life as a disabled person.

Unexpected Death of a Loved One

The untimely loss of a loved one often triggers shock, disbelief, anger, guilt, anxiety, and depression. Nightmares and loss of sleep, loss of appetite, fatigue, weight gain or loss, social withdrawal, and disinterest in things that you'd previously enjoyed are also signs of the incredible stress that such a crisis can trigger. And it might seem like these feelings and behaviors will never let up. But these experiences are part of *grief*—a normal and natural response to tragic loss. Everyone grieves a little differently, depending on factors such as the nature of the loss, personality and coping style, and previous life experiences.

Lots of people have misconceptions about grief and the grieving process—misconceptions that lead to stress because they involve black-and-white and catastrophic thinking (along with other stress-provoking thinking patterns). That's why it's important to understand grief and the grieving process. Doing so will help keep your stress in check while you're grieving. Read the following statements and mark each one as true or false by circling the choice you think is correct:

1. Grief should last about a year.   True   False

2. It's important to be strong in the face of a loss.   True   False

3. If you don't cry, it means you aren't truly sorry about the loss.   True   False

4. The grief feelings will go away if you ignore them.   True   False

Did you mark any of these statements as true? The fact is that they're all false. There's no right or wrong time frame for grieving. While it's true that most people start to feel better after weeks or months, for others it can be years. Feeling sad, frightened, or lonely is a normal reaction to loss. You don't need to put up a brave front or be afraid to show others how you feel. In fact, showing your true feelings can be very helpful. And while crying is a common response to sadness and loss, it's not the *only* one. If you don't cry, you've probably got other ways of experiencing and showing the pain you're in. Finally, trying to ignore or suppress your true feelings will only cause you more stress in the long run. Facing your grief and actively dealing with it are the best ways to heal. Finally, the feelings of grief can seem scary. You might be worried they'll last forever or spiral out of control until you "lose it" or "go crazy." But as mentioned before, these are normal and temporary experiences that typically lift with time.

Probably the most important factor in keeping your stress levels in check after a tragic loss is having the support of other people. Sharing your feelings of loss with others makes the burden of grief easier to bear. Whether you need help with funeral arrangements, regarding the deceased person's will, or just a shoulder to cry on, now is the time to lean on others who care about you—even if you take pride in being strong and self-sufficient. You might also find a bereavement group helpful if you're feeling lonely (you can contact local hospitals, funeral homes, and counseling centers). There's something about sharing your grief experiences with others who are going through similar circumstances. Finally, talking to a counselor or therapist specializing in grief and bereavement can be helpful.

While this chapter covers the basics of how to manage grief following a tragic loss, there are entire books on this subject that include more detail. The Resources (pages 317–318) list some that include self-help materials. Probably the best way to prevent problems with complicated grief is to seek professional help and get support from friends and family. Grief counseling can help you accept your loss, identify and express your feelings (for example, anger, guilt, anxiety, helplessness, and sadness), adapt to life without the person who died (for example, making decisions alone), begin new relationships, and get through important times such as birthdays and anniversaries, and can provide continuous support.

JOB LOSS

Stress from job loss is complex because it's triggered by both emotional and practical issues. You're left with a range of negative emotions—loss of self-worth, lack of a sense of control, and so on—and, of course, the financial concerns and need to look for a new job. While it's perfectly reasonable to be affected by stress at a time like this, you can keep things in check using a combination of stress management techniques, as we'll see in just a bit.

*After losing a job it's normal to go through stages of **denial**, **anger**, **frustration**, and eventually **adaptation** as you come to grips with the emotional and practical matters and move on with life.*

Consider Denise, who was the breadwinner of her family. She was laid off unexpectedly when the research firm she worked for downsized and dismissed most of her department. At first she was in denial—"This can't really be happening to me." But when the reality of having to clean out her office finally hit, she felt a combination of anger and depression. Then came the anxiety: How would she provide for her family? What about health insurance coverage? Would she be able to find a new job?

What techniques would you suggest Denise use to manage the stress of losing her job? Prioritize the seven techniques listed next (first, second, third, and so forth—you don't have to use all of them) and briefly describe to the right how Denise might use each. Read on to see what Denise actually did.

_____ Problem solving: _____

_____ Communication/assertiveness: _____

_____ Time management: _____

_____ Cognitive therapy: _____

_____ Muscle relaxation: _____

_____ Meditation: _____

_____ Healthy lifestyle: _____

Dealing with Negative Emotions

Her first day at home, Denise threw herself into a job search online. But her attention was scattered, her heart kept pounding when she saw how few jobs were out there in her field, and she periodically felt like just crawling back into bed. She couldn't imagine presenting herself to a prospective employer as a confident, competent worker. So she turned back to Chapter 8 to identify and modify the thinking patterns leading to her stressful negative emotions. She began by keeping track of these feelings and emotions over a few days and, not surprisingly, found that her levels of depression, anger, and anxiety were high. Like many people who lose their jobs, Denise had the following stress-inducing cognitions that were fueling her emotions:

Cognitions Leading to Depression

- "I'm such a loser."

- "I'm not worthwhile."

- "I should have seen this coming."

- "It's not fair."

- "I could have done more to prevent this."

Cognitions Leading to Anger

- "They don't respect me."

- "They're bastards for firing me!"

Cognitions Leading to Anxiety and Worry

- "I'll never find as good a job as that one."

- "I won't be able to support my family."

- "What if I don't find another job or earn enough money?"

Next Denise analyzed these cognitions using the strategies in Chapter 8 to come up with more logical, stress-reducing ways of thinking. Using the worksheets in that chapter, she could see that she'd lost her job because of the recession, not because of something she did. She also reminded herself that she still had her personal strengths as a worker, parent, wife, and friend. Accepting the layoff and concentrating on her strengths lifted the depressive emotions and prepared her to look for another job with renewed confidence. When she tried putting herself in her employer's shoes, she realized it wasn't a manager's personal flaw or lack of respect for her that had led to her firing; it was circumstances beyond everyone's control. Thinking this way helped Denise see that she was annoyed at the *situation*, but not furious at particular *people*—an angry, resentful state that was robbing her of valuable energy. To challenge her anxiety, Denise reminded herself that she had always saved money in a "rainy day fund" so that her family wouldn't go broke in case of an emergency such as this; and that she was extremely qualified— she'd find work, even if it wasn't her dream job. Rather than feeling so *anxious*, Denise emerged from working on her cognitions appropriately *concerned*, but ready to tackle the practical issues that lay ahead.

During this crisis, Denise also turned to meditation—something she'd never tried before. With some help from Chapter 9, as well as the daily class she started attending, she took to quieting her mind this way. Meditating became a routine that helped Denise with the stress in her life in a healthy way. She also made sure to keep up with her exercising. Previously, Denise exercised with her coworkers at lunch by taking walks. After thinking about it, she decided to change her routine and join the fitness club where her husband and son worked out several times each week. Denise soon found exercising first thing in the morning to be an excellent stress reducer that also gave her a surge of energy for tackling what were unavoidably trying days.

Taking Care of the Practical Stuff

After about a week of working on stress-reducing thinking patterns, Denise began to get some perspective on her situation, and her initial wave of intense stress started to dissipate. Between this and her meditation practice, she felt she was now in the proper frame of mind to take care of the important practical matters that needed attending to. She used the problem-solving techniques in Chapter 5 and began by listing the issues that needed to be taken care of. Her problem list appears at the bottom of the page.

It seemed obvious to Denise that getting a new job should be her number-one priority. But it could take time, and the task felt overwhelming at first. So she looked into unemployment benefits first. Planning how to meet the Department of Labor criteria for receiving benefits made her feel like she had taken an important step toward at least temporary financial security. Likewise, she investigated how to purchase temporary health insurance at a group rate through COBRA (the Consolidated Omnibus Budget Reconciliation Act). This eased some of her worry about potential medical expenses.

The prospect of a significant change in lifestyle can be stress inducing in and of itself, but Denise found next that uncovering ways to cut costs wasn't as onerous as it had seemed. Using cell phones and getting rid of their landline, switching to the least expensive cable TV package, buying food in bulk, and eliminating dining out for the time being weren't major sacrifices and made the whole family feel like they were working together to deal with the crisis.

Because of its many possible effects on a family's life, the loss of a job can seem like an overwhelming problem to deal with. That's why the best way to reduce the accompanying stress is to take a systematic, step-by-step approach to tackling one issue at a time, identifying what you can do quickly and easily to have a measurable impact first, as Denise did. Throwing yourself frantically into a chaotic job search may not be the best move.

Denise's problem solving, particularly her brainstorming, proved particularly fruitful when it came to locating sources of income. Besides getting free advice from a job recruiter friend about her résumé, Denise explored other ways of earning money on the side. For example, the old clothes that she'd planned to take to Goodwill she instead sold at a garage sale. Denise also had excellent editorial skills, so she placed flyers at local high schools and universities to see if she could earn some money helping students with their papers. She helped out with her husband's freelancing as a photographer, Web designer, and golf instructor. Specifically, Denise took care of tasks that would allow her husband

---

Denise's Problem List

1. *I need to find another job or make some money.*

2. *Do I qualify for unemployment compensation?*

3. *I have to make sure the family has health insurance while I'm out of work.*

4. *We need to reduce how much money we spend.*

to be more productive with his work and earn more money. Although the money she brought in as a result of these activities paled in comparison to what she would make in a full-time job, working hard and doing her part while she waited to hear from potential employers helped reduce Denise's stress level. Even though it took her several months to find a new permanent position, her stress never spun out of control because she could see the fruits of all of her other efforts around her every day.

WORKSHEET: PREPARING FOR A POSSIBLE LAYOFF

Do you stress out about being laid off? In this economic environment, you're not alone. But you can reduce your anxiety if you're prepared just in case the worst happens. And if you've been laid off, developing a plan might shorten how long you spend unemployed. Use this worksheet to help you.

- **Networking:** List ideas for making new contacts and exchanging ideas—for example, using social media such as Facebook.

- **Your résumé:** Is it updated? What new skills, milestones, and projects can you add?

- **Keep learning:** How can you polish up your skills or hone new ones?

14

Living a Stress-Less Lifestyle

I hope that as a result of learning about how stress works and practicing the techniques in this workbook you've been able to begin reducing the degree of stress in your life, whether that means solving problems and communicating more effectively, changing stress-inducing thoughts, or building up your stress resistance with meditation, relaxation, or tension-diffusing exercise. In this chapter, we'll shift the focus of your work from *learning* stress management techniques to *keeping* stress at bay by maintaining a stress-less lifestyle. You'll learn how long-term stress management is not a single event but rather an ongoing process.

Stress doesn't take breaks, and neither should you when it comes to practicing and using stress management tools.

Have you ever decided to go on a diet to lose weight? Many people who realize they're overweight and need to change their eating habits think, "I'll just go on a diet for a month or two to take off the extra pounds." But there's a problem: diets are like a light switch: *click!*—you're on a diet; *click!*—you're off a diet. As soon as the diet ends, your old eating habits return along with the weight you lost. Diets can be good short-term solutions for weight loss, but they often fail in the long run. It's the same with managing stress. Lasting triumph over stressors requires you to adopt a lifestyle of using the tools that you've learned here. To put it simply, stress management is an ongoing and lifelong process.

In this chapter you'll learn to think of the strategies and techniques in this workbook as a permanent *lifestyle change*. I'll help you set goals for long-term stress management and stay alert for setbacks that can derail your attempts to achieve these goals. I'll also help you cultivate a mindset and routine to make you more resilient to the

If staying healthy and in control of stress is your end goal, then your end goal really has no end. It's a lifelong goal. You have to keep using the anti-stress techniques, because that's what a healthy person does.

negative impact of stress. Think of it this way: finishing this workbook is actually the *beginning*—not the *end*—of your anti-stress journey.

MEASURING YOUR PROGRESS: AN ONGOING PROCESS

Since stress management is an ongoing process, assessing your improvement should be ongoing as well. Back in Chapter 1 you completed the Perceived Stress Scale and I suggested completing this questionnaire every month or so to track your progress. This helps you stay aware of how hard you have to work and where you need to focus your efforts. If you've been tracking your progress this way, that's great. If not, now is a good time to retake the scale and see how your score differs from when you started using the skills you've learned in this workbook. The instructions for completing the questionnaire, computing your score, and understanding what it means appear on pages 8–10. If you like, you can even figure out your percentage change by entering your scores into the following formula:

Beginning score – Current score ÷ Beginning score = Percent change

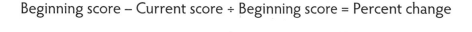

 Don't be discouraged if you're not happy with your score or how big your changes have been. The thing about managing stress is that there will always be more chances to practice the techniques. And the more you practice, the better you'll get at using these tools. Remember to keep up with monthly assessments to monitor your progress.

SETTING AND ACHIEVING STRESS MANAGEMENT GOALS

"If you aim at nothing, you will surely hit it." This simple yet inspirational adage captures the importance of setting goals for managing stress. Imagine you're playing basketball and you've got the ball. You jump and shoot the ball, but wait . . . there's no basket! To win at basketball, you have to make more baskets than the other team. So when there's no basket, there's no way of knowing if you've won the game, right? It's the same thing with stress management. You need to have a target—a goal—that helps you measure success. In this section, I'll help you set goals for continuing to use the stress management techniques over the longer term.

Setting SMART Goals

Goal setting is the process of deciding on (1) what's important for you to achieve and (2) in what time frame you want to achieve it. But not all goals that people set for themselves are effective. I recommend using the acronym SMART to help you decide on goals that will keep you working hard at implementing the techniques in this workbook. In particular, your goals should be:

S = Specific

M = Measurable

A = Achievable

R = Relevant/realistic

T = Time bound

Specific

Think of your goals as your road map to success. They need to be as detailed and specific as possible. State exactly what you want to achieve. This will help you focus your efforts and clearly define what you're striving to do. For example, if you were trying to become more fit, the goal of "getting in better shape" would be too vague. It would be more helpful to set a specific goal, such as "join a health club and hire a trainer this week," or "spend 30 minutes a day on aerobic exercise." In stress management terms, simply saying "My goal is to manage stress" or "I want to get more out of life" is not enough. The box below contains examples of specific stress-management goals.

One thing you might have noticed about the goals listed in the box is that they're all based on personal performance. Setting *performance goals* allows *you* to determine whether you meet your goals. *Outcome goals*, on the other hand, are based on the rewards of achieving something. Maybe less stress means you end up with healthier relationships with others, but with outcome goals you can't always depend on others (or on situations) to give you rewards. For example, what if you use assertiveness skills with your boss, but he still doesn't give you that raise you're asking for? If you had set an outcome goal of "getting a raise" (which requires your boss's approval), then you would not meet your goal. But if you set a performance goal of "using assertive communication to ask for a raise," you would have achieved the goal and could draw satisfaction and self-confidence from your success.

Sample Specific Goals for Managing Stress

- Spend at least 30 minutes exercising 5 days a week.
- Use problem-solving strategies to make decisions.
- Use *I* statements when expressing disappointment.
- Think and behave assertively rather than passively.
- Reduce time spent on minor, less important, tasks.
- Use cognitive therapy strategies to challenge stressful thinking patterns.
- Spend 20 minutes meditating 5 days a week.
- Use the bed only for sleep and sexual activity.

> ### Outcome Goals versus Noticing Outcome
>
> There's a difference between *setting* outcome goals—which can be problematic—and *noticing* your outcome or improvement when you use stress management strategies. For example, the Perceived Stress Scale is a way of measuring your outcome. But setting a goal of lowering your score on this scale by a certain amount can be problematic because you might not have control over some factors that go into your score. On the other hand, it's entirely worthwhile to use the Perceived Stress Scale to monitor changes in your stress levels (that is, your outcome) as a result of setting and achieving performance goals.

Measurable

Goals also need to be measurable so that you know when you've succeeded. So choose concrete goals you can easily keep track of. The examples on the previous page all adhere to this rule. "I will spend 20 minutes each day meditating," for example, gives a specific target to be measured (in this case, with a clock): time spent meditating. On the other hand, "I want to control my stress" is not a measurable goal: how will you decide when you've got *control*?

Achievable

Your goals should challenge you to stay focused and committed to using the stress-reduction techniques, but at the same time they need to be realistic. If you set goals that stretch you slightly—that require *some* effort to achieve—you'll feel like you can achieve them and stay motivated. On the other hand, you probably won't stay committed to goals you set that are too far out of reach. For example, "I will never procrastinate again" is probably unattainable, especially if you're just beginning to work on managing your time. When you eventually realize trying for such a goal is a lost cause, you'll feel demoralized and risk losing momentum. Instead, "I will use anti-procrastination strategies to help get the housework done on time this week" is probably a more reasonable (and also a more *specific*) goal. Don't bite off more than you can chew!

On the other hand, be careful not to set goals *too* low. Aim for goals that are *just out of reach*. When you accomplish one, you'll have the momentum to move on to another. Many people with stress, for instance, aim to improve their time management over 1 month, work on assertiveness communication the following month, and then add meditation to their routine the month after that. The eventual result is a dramatic decrease in stress; but they've broken it down into smaller, achievable goals (steps) rather than trying to do it all at once. Think about it; if it takes you 15 minutes to run 1 mile but you want to be able to run it in 7 minutes, you wouldn't expect to cut your time down all at once (this would be next to impossible). Instead, you would first aim for 14 minutes, then for 13, 12, and so on until you could run the mile in 7 minutes. Try to apply the same strategy to working on reducing stress. When you pick achievable goals, you figure out new ways to reach them. This, along with being successful, helps you stay motivated. In time, your smaller achievements add up and you will be able to look back at how far you've come.

Relevant

Without some sort of emotional tie to your goals, you'll have trouble keeping up the motivation to achieve them. In other words, your goals should mean something to you—they should be *relevant*. If you're working on managing stress, they should obviously relate to success with this problem. Of course, this doesn't rule out striving for goals in related areas such as work (I will delegate more tasks to others) or family life (I'll use assertiveness strategies with my mother-in-law this Thanksgiving). However, make sure you stick to performance goals rather than outcome goals. Tying goals to something that's important to you will build your commitment to achieving it. To ensure that a goal is relevant, ask yourself how achieving it will affect your overall success in controlling stress and your quality of life.

Time Bound

Finally, your goals should have a time frame. That is, you need a start date and an end date, for example, "by the end of the day," "in 1 week," or "in 3 months." By putting an end point on your goal you make it a priority, which increases motivation. Goals without specific time frames are less likely to be met because you feel you can put them off. As with goals in general, the time frame you choose should be realistic. It should also be fairly short-term. Setting short-term goals will keep you active in your battle against stress. Long-term goals (more than a few weeks) don't provide the same sense of urgency and motivation to start taking action as short-term goals do. Here are some examples of short-term goals:

- "I will buy and begin using a day planner tomorrow to keep track of my appointments."

- "I will schedule an appointment with a trainer at the gym this week."

- "I will spend 30 minutes a day using cognitive restructuring techniques."

- "I will use problem-solving techniques to deal with my neighbor on Thursday."

- "I will read food labels at the grocery store when I go shopping today."

Choosing *Your* Goals

Keeping the SMART guidelines in mind, take some time to think about what you want to achieve for yourself. Think about the following:

- Why did you buy this book?

- What would you like to change about how you manage stress?

- How does stress interfere with your life?

- What do you have to gain by reducing your stress?

- What negative consequences of stress would you like to remove from your life?

Actually writing down your goals greatly increases your chances of success. Simply thinking about them is not enough. The worksheet on the next page contains questions to help you think carefully about your goals. I recommend making copies of the blank form so you can use it for additional sets of goals. There is also little point in setting goals unless you *review* them on a regular basis—*weekly* is good; *daily* is better!—to monitor and steer your progress. Post your written goals where you can easily see them: the refrigerator, your mirror, your desk. On page 301 is a sample Personal Goals for Managing Stress form that was completed by Candice, who worked in a human resources department within a large university and had problems with work stress, as well as the stresses of raising a young family.

Rewarding Yourself

Don't fall into the trap of trying to get motivated by making yourself feel guilty or ashamed. Never beat yourself up about the problems you haven't overcome yet. Imagine trying to motivate other people this way. Do you think they'd stick around? How successful would they be?

Instead of focusing on what you haven't yet accomplished, reward yourself each time you achieve one of your goals. Giving yourself a pat on the back and a word of encouragement will not only make you feel good but will motivate you to work even harder toward your next goal. Even the smallest of rewards can work wonders as you move from goal to goal. Think about how you'll reward yourself for accomplishing each of your goals (there is space on the Personal Goals for Managing Stress worksheet for writing down your reward system). Make your rewards meaningful and pleasurable to you (see Candice's examples, as well as some more below). Use smaller rewards for meeting smaller goals and bigger ones after you've accomplished larger goals over the longer term. Create a celebration that you can anticipate and then keep it within sight all the time. Finally, be honest with yourself. Fudging the numbers mentally, or "borrowing" against the next reward, will hurt you in the long run. Remember to keep your focus on reducing stress, not just figuring out how to get the reward. If you need help thinking of rewards, some examples my patients have used are in the Eye Opener on page 302.

Your willingness to work hard at managing stress might waver over time. When the going gets rough, you can help sustain your motivation by reviewing your goals. Luckily, one advantage of the techniques I describe in Part II is that the more you use them, the more successfully you'll be able to use them. Getting started is often the hardest

PERSONAL GOALS FOR MANAGING STRESS

My personal goals for managing stress are:

1. _____

2. _____

3. _____

4. _____

5. _____

What made me choose these goals? Why are they important to me?

It's important for me to reduce my stress because . . .

1. _____

2. _____

3. _____

4. _____

5. _____

If I work hard on managing stress, my life is likely to change in the following ways:

1. _____

2. _____

3. _____

4. _____

5. _____

If I do *not* work on stress, the following negative things could happen:

1. _____

2. _____

3. _____

4. _____

5. _____

When I accomplish each goal, I will reward myself with . . .

1. _____

2. _____

3. _____

4. _____

5. _____

PERSONAL GOALS FOR MANAGING STRESS: CANDICE

My personal goals for managing stress are:

1. _Meet all of my deadlines at work_

2. _Communicate more assertively with coworkers and other people I interact with at work_

3. _Work out a more satisfying schedule with my husband for supervising the children_

4. _Practice meditation for at least 30 minutes 5 days each week_

5. _____

What made me choose these goals? Why are they important to me?

It's important for me to reduce my stress because . . .

1. _I'm feeling burnt out at work._

2. _I want to show my coworkers that I'm stronger than they think I am._

3. _I don't want to argue with my husband about who's watching the kids._

4. _I don't know which I dread more: going to work or coming home at the end of the day!_

5. _____

If I work hard on managing stress, my life is likely to change in the following ways:

1. _I will feel more confident at work._

2. _I'll feel better about communicating with department chairs, even when I have to tell them things they don't want to hear._

3. _Better relationships with family (husband, kids)_

4. _I'll feel better about going home at the end of the day._

5. _I won't have problems with lateness._

If I do *not* work on stress, the following negative things could happen:

1. _I'll continue to feel burnt out and become less productive at work._

2. _I'll dread meeting with department chairs and procrastinate._

3. _I'll keep missing deadlines._

4. _My marriage will suffer._

5. _____

When I accomplish each goal, I will reward myself with . . .

1. _After each day that I use assertive communication, I will take a nice bubble bath that evening._

2. _After I complete an assignment on time, I will treat myself to a massage._

3. _When I reduce my scores, I will buy the laptop computer I've been saving up for._

4. _____

5. _____

EYE OPENER
Real Rewards Chosen by Real People

- Take a vacation or weekend getaway.

- Put $1 in a jar every time you meet a goal. When it gets to $50, treat yourself.

- See a movie.

- Buy a new CD or DVD.

- Go for a spa treatment or massage.

- Buy yourself a gift certificate.

- Take a limo ride.

- Subscribe to a magazine you always wanted.

- Watch your favorite TV show.

- Enjoy a nice meal at a fancy restaurant.

- Buy something for your hobby.

- Find some time to be by yourself.

- Pay someone to do the yard work or house cleaning this week.

part—and there will be occasional bumps in the road ahead—but for the most part, your successes in helping yourself will provide ongoing motivation.

MAKING STRESS MANAGEMENT TECHNIQUES A PERMANENT PART OF YOUR LIFESTYLE

When you practice something over and over, and work it into your routine, it becomes part of your *lifestyle*. In other words, something you just *do* without needing to think too much about it. Take brushing your teeth as an example. You don't ask yourself if you *need* to brush your teeth. You simply do it (probably more than once each day) without too much effort or struggle. If you're going to keep your stress levels under control over the long haul and meet the goals you've set out for yourself, then you'll need to make the stress management techniques part of your routine—your lifestyle. Here are some suggestions for how.

Work Stress Management into Your Schedule

The most straightforward way to make sure you're incorporating stress management techniques into your routine is to schedule them into your day (for example, using your daily planner). That is, make a "date" with yourself and treat it as seriously as you would a doctor's appointment, important work meeting, or dinner date. If it seems like there aren't enough hours in the day already, use the time management strategies in Chapter 7 to help you make time for stress management. And consider the time you set aside to practice these skills an investment: Putting in the time up front will pay you dividends in terms of increased energy, productivity, and mental clarity down the road. You'll actually be more productive when you spend time working on stress management.

It might seem like you don't have the time to invest in practicing stress management skills right now, but when you're less stressed you'll more than make up for it.

Anita scheduled going to the gym into her daily routine on her way home from work. Within a week she was hooked and had even made a new friend there, whom she started working out and socializing with. Bart set aside his lunch break every other day to practice cognitive therapy techniques. He'd work through some of the forms in Chapter 8 while he sat in his office and play enjoyable music in the background. Clive set his alarm a half hour earlier in the morning so he could get up, take a hot shower, and spend time meditating before leaving for work.

How can you schedule regular "appointments" with yourself to practice working on stress management? Fill in your own ideas in the form on the next page and then make sure to add them to your daily planner. Many e-mail programs and smartphones allow you to send yourself automatic reminders for certain activities when the time to do them rolls around. If possible, use these features to ensure that you don't overlook your stress management practice time.

Use Prompts and Reminders

Just as the alarm clock prompts you to get out of bed in the morning, and the note you wrote to yourself last night reminds you to give your daughter two dollars to buy her lunch at school today, you can use prompts and reminders to kick-start stress management routines. Ellen, for example, decided to practice relaxation strategies for 30 minutes every night as soon as she got into bed. At first she had to remind herself with a sticky note on the night table that simply read "relaxation!" but after a few days it became a habit—automatic—a routine that she hardly had to think about doing at all.

The best cues and reminders are those that occur naturally and frequently. Some examples are hanging up the telephone, eating, driving, turning off the TV, and the like. Whenever these things happen, follow them with a certain stress management technique: diaphragmatic breathing, relaxation, meditation, using cognitive therapy, thinking of something assertive to say to someone, and so on. At first you might need extra reminders to follow these new "rules," but if you're consistent, they'll become habits that you'll automatically do. Take a few minutes to set up five rules to help you stick with your stress management lifestyle. Some examples appear on the next page.

SCHEDULING STRESS MANAGEMENT PRACTICE

Day	Time	Stress management activity to practice

- Every time you turn off a light switch, take note of your breathing pattern and breathe diaphragmatically.

- Whenever you throw something in a trash can, notice the tension in your shoulders and practice brief relaxation strategies.

- Practice listening skills during TV commercials.

- Use your time in the shower to think about any stressful thought patterns and how you could challenge and modify them.

Now write your new rules in the spaces provided in the worksheet at the top of page 305.

Seize the Moment

Another way to help make stress management techniques part of your routine is to get in the habit of taking advantage of "downtime" to practice your strategies. Sitting in the dentist's chair? Why not practice diaphragmatic breathing? Riding on a bus, train, or plane? Why not try out cognitive therapy or work through some problem solving? At a social event? Practice effective communication strategies such as giving compliments (assertiveness) and listening carefully. Waiting in traffic or in line at the store (or anywhere else)? These are great opportunities to practice muscle relaxation or meditation. The goal of sneaking in some practice with the anti-stress strategies while you're in different situations is to prepare you for when you'll need to call on them while you're on the go. Complete the Opportunities to Practice Stress Management Techniques worksheet at the bottom of page 305 by coming up with situations and methods you can practice.

MY PROMPTS AND REMINDERS FOR PRACTICING STRESS MANAGEMENT

1. _____

2. _____

3. _____

4. _____

5. _____

Put Life on Hold . . . Occasionally

Getting away from it all and taking a nice long vacation—a week at the beach, 2 weeks overseas—can be a terrific way to get some rest and relaxation. But beware of two disadvantages of lengthy vacations. The first is that things seem to pile up when you're away for so long, so that by the end of your first day back in your regular routine it feels like you never left—like you need another vacation! Which leads to the second downside: because you're probably able to take only one or two major vacations each year, your next break might be months away. That's why, for your anti-stress lifestyle, I recommend building in more frequent, but shorter, getaways such as half-day or full-day trips, overnights, long weekends, and so on. Spread these mini-vacations out over the course of the year (perhaps once a month) and you'll always have something enjoyable to look forward

OPPORTUNITIES TO PRACTICE STRESS MANAGEMENT TECHNIQUES

Situation	Techniques to practice
1.	
2.	
3.	
4.	
5.	

to in the near future. This alone will help you destress. Not to mention the benefits of getting out of your routine and enjoying more fun and rewarding activities.

Schedule Time to Get Away

What's that you're saying to yourself? You'd like to get away, but your life is so stressful and there's never a good time? That's exactly the reason you need mini-vacations—to take some of the pressure off. And if you're waiting for the perfect time to get away, good luck. There won't ever be a *perfect* time—you'll be waiting forever. If you're thinking this way, it might also be a sign that you could benefit from Chapter 7 on time management.

If you're going to be committed to a stress-reducing lifestyle, you'll need to be *proactive* (think assertive) about your schedule. This means sitting down with your planner and scheduling your getaways (including requesting the time off from work) months in advance so that you can stick to your plans. Plan several of these mini-vacations at the same time and remember to spread your actual trips (or time off) out over the course of the year. That way, they're already in your planner and you won't find yourself reacting to a schedule that's imposed on you.

Keep a Vacation Folder

Once you've planned to get away for short jaunts several times a year, you'll need to think about where to go and what to do on your getaways. Sure, a day on the golf course, shopping mall, or beach will be terrific; but you'll need other options for when the weather doesn't cooperate or if these activities become repetitive. That's why I suggest starting a folder or file of information about places you can get away to quickly. You might find that there are lots of interesting places within a few hours' drive (or a short flight) from home. Put in your folder notes from friends about their trips, brochures, newspaper and magazine clippings, and information you print off from the Internet. Go to the bookstore and the library, and go online to read about day trips in your area. Include everything you find in your file. That way, when you're looking for something interesting to try, you'll have all sorts of options at your fingertips.

Here are some examples of getaways that my patients have told me about: trying out a new golf course in another part of the state, spending a night at a bed and breakfast inn in a nearby city or town, touring vineyards and wineries, spending a night in an extravagant hotel/spa, or visiting a nearby apple or berry orchard. You probably have ideas of your own (you can start a list in the spaces that follow). If not, start building your vacation folder!

Ideas for One- or Two-Day Getaways

_____

_____

_____

_____

_____

_____

TROUBLESHOOTING

Keeping up with managing stress over the long term isn't easy. And the thought that you need to make these strategies part of your permanent lifestyle might even seem daunting. As they become part of your routine, things won't seem as difficult. Yet if you're having trouble staying motivated to continue, the worksheet on the next page can help:

Another trouble spot to avoid is setting rigid or absolutist goals. Alejandro, for example, set an unrealistic goal for himself: he declared that he'd meditate *every day this month*. But this is like setting yourself up for failure. Inevitably, you're going to miss a day for one reason or another. One day, when Alejandro simply didn't feel like meditating, he started beating up on himself: "I have no self-control." This led to more stress and other maladaptive thoughts, such as "Now that I've broken my rule, it doesn't even matter if I meditate." That's when things really started going downhill.

You can't expect perfection when it comes to managing stress. Occasional slips, like the one Alejandro had, are completely normal. And they're not caused by a lack of willpower. Usually they arise from certain situations or events or because of a lack of practice. Fortunately, all of these things are controllable. The *abstinence violation effect* occurs when you set an unrealistic rule for yourself. Once you break your rule, it starts to seem like it's okay to keep breaking the rule. This leads you in the wrong direction. To avoid falling into this trap, don't be a perfectionist. Expect that from time to time you'll experience some stress. But remember that you know what to do about it.

What If You're Not Where You Want to Be?

Getting the upper hand on stress is no small task, so your progress might be slower than you'd hoped for. If you feel you have achieved all you can achieve using the tools in this book but the yardsticks you're using to gauge your success indicate you're still under a lot of stress, don't despair. Instead, take some time to pinpoint the strategies that have worked best for you. You might be able to further reduce your stress if you concentrate more on these.

Read through the Stress Management Strategies Checklist on page 310 and mark the tools that you've found most effective. In addition, think about what you've learned by using these strategies and fill out the Stress Management Review worksheet on page 311. You might find it useful to repeat these exercises in the weeks and months to come as you hone your awareness of what works best for you, so make extra copies of both forms.

STAYING MOTIVATED

- Make a list of the benefits of continuing to use stress management strategies. How will they help improve your family or work life? Your social activities? How will working on reducing stress affect the way you view yourself?

  _____

  _____

  _____

- How will your performance improve in the areas of life you value (such as work, home, school, social life, volunteer work, recreation)?

  _____

  _____

  _____

  _____

  _____

  _____

- How will your self-image improve?

  _____

  _____

  _____

  _____

- Thinking about your personal progress can be very motivating. How are things better now, compared to when you began using this workbook? Note this below.

  _____

  _____

  _____

(cont.)

STAYING MOTIVATED (cont.)

- Choose a specific short-term goal and a reward for achieving this goal. Make sure you reward your-self only when you reach the goal. Record your goals and rewards on the form below.

- Make a contract with yourself where you agree to enjoy certain activities (watching a movie, taking a trip, making a large purchase) only after you've practiced certain stress management strategies for an entire week. Fill in this information on the form further down on this page.

Goal:

_____

_____

_____

To be achieved by: /   /   [insert date]

Reward for reaching the goal by the deadline:

_____

_____

_____

For 1 week, starting on   /   /   [insert date], I will:

_____

_____ [insert a specific stress management technique to practice every day of the week].

If I don't reach my week's goal, I will not:

_____

_____ [insert a desirable activity, purchase, or other event that you will deny yourself at the end of the week unless you meet your week's goal].

STRESS MANAGEMENT STRATEGIES CHECKLIST

	Chapter	Strategy
1. _____	5	Problem solving
2. _____	6	Building assertiveness skills
3. _____	6	Anti-stress listening and speaking
4. _____	7	Time management
5. _____	7	Getting organized
6. _____	7	Reducing procrastination
7. _____	8	Cognitive therapy (recognizing, challenging, and modifying stress-provoking thoughts)
8. _____	9	Diaphragmatic breathing
9. _____	9	Progressive muscle relaxation/brief relaxation
10. _____	9	Mantra meditation
11. _____	9	Mindfulness mediation
12. _____	10	Healthy eating habits
13. _____	10	Exercising
14. _____	10	Sleeping well

From *The Stress Less Workbook*. Copyright 2012 by The Guilford Press.

DEALING WITH LAPSES AND PREVENTING RELAPSES

Even if you're working hard at maintaining a stress-less lifestyle, there will be bumps in the road. And when you hit one of these bumps, you'll need to step it up to keep from backsliding into old stress-inducing patterns. It's important that you not let these temporary setbacks turn into a full-blown return of your old ways. This requires understanding the differences between lapses and relapses and knowing how to deal with the former before they become the latter.

What Is a *Lapse*?

Simply put, a lapse is a slip—a noticeable increase in your stress levels after you've started making progress toward reducing stress. And realizing that a lapse is occurring can be tricky because the first signs are not always feelings of anxiety and worry. Physical symptoms such as trouble sleeping, increased muscle tension, reduced appetite or sex drive, and recurring headaches might be the first warning signs of your lapse. Behavioral signs, such as anger, irritability, or an increase in avoidance might also be what tip you off. Take Judith, for example, who was stressed about how the struggling economy would affect the family's business. She'd made great strides in reducing stress and was finally sleeping better and putting on the weight she'd lost over the past year. But one evening, Judith's husband pointed out that every night that week she'd been having arguments with their 12-year-old daughter and waking up in the middle of the night to get extra work done. These were the first signals that Judith was experiencing a lapse. But a lapse might have less obvious signs. C. J., for example, had worked hard to overcome his constant stressing about his aging parents, who were now ill. Then he found himself skipping his daily gym visits and instead coming home from work and sleeping for a few hours before dinner.

You may be thinking that I'm making a big deal out of nothing. Perhaps Judith's concerns were justified—the family business, after all, was taking a financial hit. Maybe C. J. was just putting in some long days at work and was too tired to go to the gym. Granted, there may be a variety of explanations for Judith's and C. J.'s behavior. On the other hand, any sign of increased stress could also point to a lapse that needs prompt attention.

STRESS MANAGEMENT REVIEW

The stress management strategies that worked best for me were:

These strategies seemed to work because:

These strategies worked best for defeating these problems:

Lapse versus Relapse

Lapses are not by themselves cause for too much alarm. They're usually temporary and easy to deal with if you view them as signs that you need to practice the strategies that worked best for you more often (see the worksheet on page 310). However, when lapses become frequent, and more the rule than the exception, you may be headed for a *relapse*—a much more profound return to the stressful thinking and behavior patterns that are harder to control. Most all relapses can be prevented. The important thing is to try to head off relapses by having a relapse prevention plan to help you deal with the lapses swiftly and effectively as they arise.

Developing Your Relapse Prevention Plan

Relapse prevention starts with being proactive and remaining aware of situations likely to cause stress or trigger a lapse. You also keep a lookout for warning signs and approach the lapse as a temporary setback that you know how to overcome. Then you use the skills and strategies you've learned throughout this workbook to turn things around. The following strategies can help you identify and effectively deal with lapses:

Identify "High-Risk" Periods

Since your chances of having a lapse increase when you've got more stressors in your life, you can prepare for an increase in stress and don't have to get taken by surprise. Of course, negative stressors can trigger a lapse. Have you recently lost a close relative or been having problems with a close relationship? Are work or financial pressures ramping up? But remember that positive events can also trigger stress, and therefore produce lapses. Will you be starting a new job? Getting married or having a baby? Setting out on your own for the first time? Have you received a major award or recognition? Maybe it's almost holiday time again. When you know that events like these—positive or negative—are coming up, prepare yourself for more stress. If you're ready, the lapse won't catch you off guard and you'll be equipped to take action immediately. If the stressful event happens without warning, you still have time to act, but remember that it's important to address lapses right away.

What are some high-risk stressors that you anticipate in the next few months? Note these in the worksheet on the facing page and use the skills that follow to defeat potential lapses. Make extra copies of the form so you can use it farther into the future too.

Spot the Warning Signs

Before you can prevent a relapse, you need to identify the signs that you're having a lapse. Here are some possible warning signs to look for:

- An increase in physical symptoms of stress and anxiety
- An increase in stressful thinking patterns
- Feeling more tired than usual

RELAPSE PREVENTION PLAN: MY HIGH-RISK SITUATIONS

1. _____

2. _____

3. _____

4. _____

5. _____

- Feeling more irritable or feeling down

- An increase in tension in your close relationships

When you spot these (or other) warning signs, you know it's time to swing into relapse prevention mode and use the techniques described below to stop the lapse in its tracks.

Be Realistic

You may be inclined to panic at the first sign of a lapse. But don't fall into the trap of beating up on yourself. Remember that lapses are normal and unavoidable. They occur sometimes despite your best intentions. Saying things to yourself such as "Oh no, I'm failing!" or "This is awful; I can't take this again" will only lead you into a cycle of despair and increase your stress. Instead of heaping criticism on your head, tell yourself that something has gone wrong that you need to correct. Then take action! The following coping statements might help you deal effectively with a lapse:

- "Everything's okay. This was bound to happen. Everyone has lapses."

- "I'm glad I caught this before it became a relapse. I know what I have to do now."

- "For whatever reason, I'm having some trouble with stress. I guess it means I need to work a little harder."

- "I've beaten this before. There's no reason I can't beat it again!"

Take Action

Flip back to the Stress Management Strategies Checklist on page 310, where you noted the strategies that you found most helpful. Because you've already used these skills, you can probably get back on track more quickly than you'd expect. It's almost a matter of reviewing what you already know and planning how you'll implement the techniques that worked best in the past.

SEEKING PROFESSIONAL HELP

Finding a Clinician

If your problems with stress are severe (perhaps you're suffering from PTSD) or don't respond to the self-help approach described in this workbook, consider making an appointment with a mental health treatment provider. Most likely, you'll have to look around a little before you find a qualified clinician. Most of the techniques described in this book fall into the category of cognitive-behavioral therapy (CBT). But not all therapists are familiar with or well trained in using this approach. If you're having trouble finding someone to work with, you might turn to two professional organizations that can provide you with a list of therapists in your region who have indicated that they use cognitive-behavioral approaches: the Association for Behavioral and Cognitive Therapies (*www.abct.org*), and the Anxiety and Depression Association of America (*www.adaa.org*).

You might also be able to get referral lists from your state, provincial, or regional mental health, psychological, and psychiatric associations. And if you happen to live near a major university that has a training program in psychology, or a medical school with a psychiatry department, you could call and find out if they have a clinic that offers treatment from their therapists-in-training. And don't be too concerned about working with a student therapist—especially one with experience using CBT: he or she will be closely supervised (and working hard to impress the supervisor!). Not only is the quality of their therapy often very good, but such clinics often provide services at low cost.

If you still can't find anyone with related expertise, check out the organizations and websites listed in the Resources at the back of this book. Many of these provide information on stress and/or help you find a cognitive-behavioral therapist.

SOME FINAL WORDS

Congratulations! You've come a long way. I hope the insights, information, and strategies I've included in this workbook have helped you reduce the amount of stress in your life. As you've learned, you have lots to gain in the short and long term by addressing the problems that led you to this workbook in the first place. Besides the fact that they're proven to work, one of the things I like most about the techniques is that once you practice and learn them, they're yours to keep (and use) forever. No relying on someone else's sage advice for what to do every week. No costly medication prescriptions that need refilling. You've got skills and knowledge that no one can take away from you. That's a resource you can't exhaust, especially when you apply your creative self-awareness to crafting the stress-less life that works best for you in meeting the challenges that lie ahead.

Resources

ASSOCIATIONS AND ORGANIZATIONS

United States

Academy of Cognitive Therapy (ACT)
www.academyofct.org
267-350-7683
 Referrals to certified cognitive therapists.

American Academy of Cognitive and Behavioral Psychology
www.americanacademyofbehavioralpsychology.org
330-672-7664
 Referrals to board-certified psychologists in cognitive-behavioral psychology.

American Dietetic Association
www.eatright.org
800-877-1600
 Provides scientific information about food and nutrition.

American Institute of Stress
www.stress.org
914-963-1200
 Information on many aspects of stress; "informational packets" can be purchased.

American Psychological Association
www.apa.org
800-374-2721
 Information and brochures on stress and anxiety, among other problems.

Anxiety and Depression Association of America
www.adaa.org
240-485-1001
 Information on support groups in the United States, Canada, South Africa, Mexico, Australia; listings for professionals who treat anxiety disorders in the United States, Canada, and elsewhere.

Anxiety-Panic.com
www.anxiety-panic.com/default.cfm
 A search engine for anxiety-related links.

Association for Behavioral and Cognitive Therapies (ABCT)
www.abct.org
212-647-1890
 Referrals to therapists and information about CBT.

Center for Mindfulness in Medicine, Health Care, and Society
www.umassmed.edu/cfm
Information about incorporating mindfulness-based meditation approaches into medicine.

Freedom from Fear
www.freedomfromfear.org
718-351-1717, ext. 24
National nonprofit advocacy organization for people with anxiety disorders and depression; offers information on support groups and other resources, plus newsletters, blogs, and bookstore.

International Association of Cognitive Psychotherapy
www.the-iacp.com
Referrals to cognitive therapists.

National Center for PTSD
www.ncptsd.va.gov
802-296-6300
Information on PTSD and its treatment.

Social Phobia/Social Anxiety Association
www.socialphobia.org
Information and links on social anxiety.

Canada

Anxiety Disorders Association of Canada (ADAC/ACTA)
www.anxietycanada.ca
613-722-0236
Links to other sites with referral options.

United Kingdom

Anxiety UK
www.anxietyuk.org.uk
08444 775 774
Information and referrals.

British Association for Behavioral and Cognitive Therapies
www.babcp.com
0161 797 4484
Offers "find a therapist" feature.

International Stress Management Association (ISMA)
www.isma.org.uk
0845 680 7083
Comprehensive information on stress, links to organizations on specific types of stress, such as stress at work, and other resources.

Stress Management Society
www.stress.org.uk
0808 231 3927
Fact sheets, newsletters, information on stress in the workplace, and other resources.

Australia/New Zealand

Anxiety Treatment Australia
www.anxietyaustralia.com.au
03 9819 3671 or 0419 104 284
Information on anxiety treatment options in Australia and a list of helpful resources.

Australian Association for Cognitive and Behavioral Therapies
www.aacbt.org
List of CBT practitioners.

Dietitians Association of Australia
www.daa.asn.au
61 2 628 29555
  Information about food and nutrition.

New Zealand Dietetic Association
www.dietitians.org.nz
04 473 3054
  Food and nutrition information.

BOOKS

Antony, M. M. (2004). *10 simple solutions to shyness: How to overcome shyness, social anxiety, and fear of public speaking.* Oakland, CA: New Harbinger.

Antony, M. M., Craske, M. G., and Barlow, D. H. (2006). *Mastering your fears and phobias* (2nd ed., workbook). New York: Oxford University Press.

Antony, M. M., and Norton, P. J. (2009). *The anti-anxiety workbook: Proven strategies to overcome worry, phobias, panic, and obsessions.* New York: Guilford Press.

Antony, M. M., and Swinson, R. P. (2008). *When perfect isn't good enough: Strategies for coping with perfectionism* (2nd ed.). Oakland, CA: New Harbinger.

Barlow, D. H., and Craske, M. G. (2007). *Mastery of your anxiety and panic* (4th ed., workbook). New York: Oxford University Press.

Bower, S. A., and Bower, G. H. (2004). *Asserting yourself: A practical guide for positive change* (updated ed.). Cambridge, MA: Da Capo.

Brach, T. (2004). *Radical acceptance.* New York: Bantam.

Burns, D. D. (1999). *The feeling good handbook* (rev. ed.). New York: Plume.

Christensen, A., and Jacobson, N. S. (2000). *Reconcilable differences.* New York: Guilford Press.

Clark, D. A., and Beck, A. T. (2011). *The anxiety and worry workbook: The cognitive behavioral solution.* New York: Guilford Press.

Covey, S. R. (2004). *The 7 habits of highly successful people* (rev. ed.). New York: Free Press.

Davidson, J. E., and Sternberg, R. J. (2003). *The psychology of problem solving.* Cambridge, UK: Cambridge University Press.

Ellis, A. (2001). *Overcoming destructive beliefs, feelings, and behaviors.* Amherst, NY: Prometheus Books.

Emmett, R. (2008). *Manage your time to reduce your stress: A handbook for the overworked, overscheduled, and overwhelmed.* New York: Walker.

Epstein, L., and Mardon, S. (2006). *The Harvard Medical School guide to a good night's sleep.* New York: McGraw-Hill.

Germer, C. K. (2009). *The mindful path to self-compassion: Freeing yourself from destructive thoughts and emotions.* New York: Guilford Press.

Goudey, P. (2000). *The unofficial guide to beating stress.* New York: IDG Books.

Greenberg, J. (2010). *Comprehensive stress management.* New York: McGraw-Hill.

Gyoerkoe, K. L., and Wiegartz, P. S. (2006). *10 simple solutions to worry: How to calm your mind, relax your body, and reclaim your life.* Oakland, CA: New Harbinger.

Hanh, Thich Nhat. (2009). *Living without stress or fear: Essential teachings on the true source of happiness* (audiobook). Louisville, CO: Sounds True.

Hauri, P., and Linde, S. (1996). *No more sleepless nights.* Hoboken, NJ: Wiley.

Hazlett-Stevens, H. (2005). *Women who worry too much: How to stop worry and anxiety from ruining relationships, work, and fun.* Oakland, CA: New Harbinger.

Hope, D. A., Heimberg, R. G., Juster, H. R., and Turk, C. L. (2000). *Managing social anxiety.* New York: Oxford University Press.

Kabat-Zinn, J. (1990). *Full catastrophe living: Using the wisdom of your body and mind to face stress, pain, and illness.* New York: Delta.

Kabat-Zinn, J. (1994). *Wherever you go, there you are: Mindfulness meditation in everyday life.* New York: Hyperion.

Klipper, M. Z., and Benson, H. (2000). *The relaxation response* (updated, expanded ed.). New York: Harper.

Luskin, F., and Pelletier, K. (2005). *Stress free for good: 10 scientifically proven life skills for health and happiness.* New York: Harper.

Monarth, H., and Kasse, L. (2007). *The confident speaker: Beat your nerves and communicate at your best in any situation.* New York: McGraw-Hill.

Morgenstern, J. (2004). *Time management from the inside out: The foolproof system for taking control of your schedule—and your life* (2nd ed.). New York: Holt.

Nay, W. R. (2012). *Taking charge of anger: Six steps to asserting yourself without losing control* (2nd ed.). New York: Guilford Press.

Nichols, M. P. (2009). *The lost art of listening: How learning to listen can improve relationships* (2nd ed.). New York: Guilford Press.

Orsillo, S. M., and Roemer, L. (2011). *The mindful way through anxiety.* New York: Guilford Press.

Rosenbloom, D., and Williams, M. B. (2010). *Life after trauma: A workbook for healing* (2nd ed.). New York: Guilford Press.

Salzberg, S. (2002). *Lovingkindness: The revolutionary art of happiness.* Boston: Shambhala.

Sapolsky, R. M. (2004). *Why zebras don't get ulcers* (3rd ed.). New York: Holt.

Satter, E. (1999). *Secrets of feeding a healthy family.* Madison, WI: Kelcyl Press.

Siegel, R. D. (2010). *The mindfulness solution: Everyday practices for everyday problems.* New York: Guilford Press.

Stahl, B., and Goldstein, E. (2010). *A mindfulness-based stress reduction workbook.* Oakland, CA: New Harbinger.

Willett, W. C. (2005). *Eat, drink, and be healthy: The Harvard Medical School guide to healthy eating.* New York: Free Press.

Index

About the Author

Jonathan S. Abramowitz, PhD, is Professor and Associate Chair of Psychology, Research Professor of Psychiatry, and Director of the Anxiety and Stress Disorders Clinic at the University of North Carolina at Chapel Hill. An award-winning expert on anxiety and stress-related disorders, Dr. Abramowitz is the author or editor of numerous books, including *Getting Over OCD*. He lives in Chapel Hill with his wife and two daughters.